Nurses

NURSES

The inside story
of the nursing profession

DONALD GOULD

UNWIN

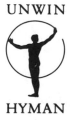

HYMAN

LONDON SYDNEY WELLINGTON

First published in Great Britain by Unwin Hyman Limited in 1988

Unwin Hyman Limited
15/17 Broadwick Street, London W1V 1FP

Allen & Unwin Australia Pty Ltd
8 Napier Street, North Sydney, NSW 2060, Australia

Allen & Unwin New Zealand Pty Ltd with Port Nicholson Press
60 Cambridge Terrace, Wellington, New Zealand

British Library Cataloguing in Publication Data

Gould, Donald
Nurses.
1. Nursing profession
I. Title
610.73'06'9

ISBN 0-04-440203-1

Printed in Great Britain by
Biddles Ltd,
Guildford and King's Lynn

CONTENTS

To nurses everywhere, and in particular to Alison Baker, Lilian Brodbin, Theresa Broderick, Marie-Louise Curtin, Clere Daly, Emma Elliott, Ruth Farrow, Steve Goodwin, Michael Jenkins, Diane Johnson, Coral Jepson, Bridget Keast-Butler, Maureen Lahiff, Martin Latham, Margaret Leader, Maggie Lyne, Ruth McArthur, Eileen Northway, Mary O'Kane', Sue Potter, Molly Pritchard, Sarah Reed, Cicely Saunders, Sue Scott, Marian Sharpe, Margaret Starkie, Anne Marie Superville and Sue Waite.

And with special thanks to John Keast-Butler, Kathleen Clarke and Jilly Rosser.

Chapter 1

INTRODUCTION

'Nurses are always portrayed as slim, blonde creatures, radiating sex appeal, but a lot of nurses I know are flat-footed, fat, and have terminal acne.'

This somewhat ungallant remark was made by a male member of the breed during one of the conversations which have provided the substance of this book. But he is no sour-spirited misogynist. He was simply attacking the highly romanticised view of nurses cherished by many and perpetuated by the kind of writers who sustain the prosperity of Mills and Boon. He wants nurses to be recognised for what they are – not 'angels in aprons' but highly-trained, hard-working, tough-minded professionals doing an essential and demanding job, often under conditions which would have your average stevedore or soldier or solicitor legging it hotfoot to the European Court of Human Rights.

Nurses sets out to do just that – to describe the nursing life as it really is by reporting, in their own words, the way a variety of labourers in the field feel about themselves and their jobs, their customers and their colleagues, including the doctors and administrators who influence their lives.

But before seeing what the workers have to say it will be useful to consider a few facts and figures which will illuminate and provide a background to their remarks.

1

FLORENCE NIGHTINGALE

Nurses of the kind we know and love are a comparatively modern invention, and Florence Nightingale is given the major credit for starting the whole thing off.

Over the centuries, and particularly since the coming of Christianity, there have always been a few high-minded individuals and groups who have devoted themselves to the physical and spiritual care of the sick. Such work was often undertaken by monks and nuns, or by military and chivalric orders such as the Knights Hospitallers of St John (male nurses have an ancient lineage, you see). But there was no widespread, organised system for the provision of nursing care. Indeed, matters got worse instead of better as time progressed, thanks largely to the Reformation.

The Lutherans and Calvinists concentrated mightily on salvation through personal faith, so that gaining Brownie points by the performance of good works became of far less importance to those hoping to earn eternal bliss, and the care of less prosperous invalids fell largely into the hands of ignorant and parasitic women who were in it for the pickings, like Sarah Gamp and Betsey Prig, portrayed in Dickens's *Martin Chuzzlewit*. Infirmaries were commonly filthy pounds in which drunken sluts stole from and abused those under their 'care'.

Florence Nightingale changed all that. The daughter of a wealthy English merchant possessed of many influential friends, she was highly educated in such unladylike fields as science, mathematics and political economy. She had no use for the sybaritic life thought appropriate to females of her class, and was determined to become an early example of the career woman.

Never one to brook obstruction, she wore down an original fierce family resistance, and left home to study and take part in the 'unsuitable' task of caring for the sick at some of the few institutions at home and abroad which, at the time, were paying any serious attention to the development of nursing as an art.

By 1854, aged 34, she had established a reputation as a forceful propagandist in the field, and was asked by the government to go to the Crimea, heading a team of 38 nursing volunteers, to organise the care of soldiers wounded in the war with Russia. She arrived to find a shambles. There were no sewers, little water, no soap, no towels and no laundry. The food was bad and the medical care desultory. Filth, lice and fleas abounded.

Not for long. This formidable woman soon had the quarter-masters and the engineers *and* the doctors doing her bidding. When she arrived the mortality rate among the wounded exceeded 50 per cent. By the time she'd got things sorted out it had fallen to 2.2 per cent.

This achievement made her a national heroine, and after her return to England in 1856 a grateful nation raised £44,000 by popular subscription, which was enough to enable her to establish a school of nursing at St Thomas' Hospital in London.

She believed that nursing should be in the hands of capable educated women who had been trained for the task, and that schools of nursing should be run by nurses and not doctors. Doctors would be paid to impart some of the substantial body of knowledge which she felt nurses needed in order to practise effectively and well, but her young ladies would not be mere handmaidens to the medical men. They would remain under the stern control of their senior member, the matron, who should be free from day-to-day interference by 'outsiders' such as physicians and hospital governors. She wanted nursing to become established as an independent profession, and, as usual, she had her way.

The Nightingale Training School opened in 1860 with an intake of 15 students. Each had a room of her own, and was given bed and board, uniform and laundering, and a suitably modest 'salary' – that is to say, a little pocket money.

The course lasted for a year, followed by a period of practice under supervision. The training was designed to enable the pupils to work in a hospital, to be capable of caring for the sick at home and to teach individuals and families how to look after themselves and avoid disease. So much for the modern conceit that health education and the value of preventive medicine are wondrous new concepts – Florence Nightingale had perceived it all.

The alumni of the Nightingale school went, or were sent, to hospitals throughout the land, spreading the gospel, and within 25 years the old-style sluttish, ignorant, self-seeking sick-attendant had virtually disappeared from the scene, to be replaced by dedicated, trained professionals.

We are all creatures of our time, and, doubtless, if Florence had never been born, somebody else, at around the same period, would have fulfilled the same role. But it happened to be her. She is the prototype of the modern nurse, and every nurse in the kingdom now is a direct descendant of the family of 15 young probationers who were the first to join her school. And nurses trained at St Thomas' are still affectionately labelled 'Nightingales'. Techniques have raced ahead of anything she can ever have imagined, but the principles of nursing she proclaimed have yet to be bettered.

Incidentally, Florence was also the first victim of the 'angels in aprons' myth. She was widely acclaimed as 'the Lady with the Lamp' because of her habit of touring the Scutari wards at night, lighting her way with a smelly oil flame, doubtless in order to make sure that all was shipshape and Bristol fashion, and that none of her nurses had skimped on the task of obeying the rules laid down. But to the wounded soldiers this nightly visitation seemed like the vision of some near-heavenly being – an 'angel of mercy', sent by the Lord to protect their lives and souls. She may, indeed, have been just that, but if so she was an angel with a strictly practical turn of mind.

She was good-looking, being possessed of the powerful kind of sex appeal which only highly intelligent women exude. She had several eminent admirers, and Benjamin Jowett, the famous master of Balliol, wanted her to be his bride.

She was witty, she was tough, she was knowledgeable, she could see what needed to be done, and she had the drive and ability to find out how to do it.

She was compassionate and entirely unsentimental.

In other words, she was your typical modern nurse.

NURSES TODAY

There are now perhaps as many as a million nurses alive and well and living in the United Kingdom, of whom some 500,000 are on the active list. Of these nearly 400,000 are employed by the National Health Service. At any one time about 300,000 NHS nurses are qualified and 100,000 are in training.

The great majority (about three-quarters) are, or are aiming to become, a so-called registered general nurse (RGN, previously called a state registered nurse or SRN), a registered mental nurse (RMN), a registered sick children's nurse (RSCN) or a registered nurse for the mentally handicapped (RNMH). All these are known collectively as first-level nurses.

A substantial minority belong to a lower caste of 'enrolled nurses'. They also may have been trained for general duties, becoming an EN/G, or for nursing the mentally ill or mentally handicapped, becoming an EN/M or EN/MH. They were previously known as, and are still commonly called, state enrolled nurses or SENs. Officially these are second-level nurses.

Qualifications for entry to the profession, the courses of instruction, the maintenance of a register, discipline, and many other matters concerning the control of nursing, are the responsibility of a statutory body called the United Kingdom Central Council for Nursing, Midwifery and Health Visiting (UKCC), which was established by the *Nurses, Midwives and Health Visitors Act* 1979. This replaced a clutch of bodies separately responsible for nursing and midwifery in the four countries of the UK. Four national boards undertake certain delegated functions.

To be accepted for training as a first-level nurse a young lady or gentleman must be at least 17 ½ years old and have achieved at least five C-grade O level passes in the examination for the General Certificate of Education, or five grade 1 passes in the Certificate of Secondary Education, or five C-level passes in the new General Certificate of Secondary Education, which has just replaced the other two. And if you can find your way through that maze of figures and initials, you're probably well qualified to join the profession. A few gain entry by passing an educational test approved by UKCC.

There then follows a three-year course of tutelage, during which the student is lectured at and works (hard) as a dogsbody on the wards and in the departments of a hospital approved as a training place. For this service she or, as it might be, he (I can't go on doing this he/she thing, so from now on I'll just say 'she' when talking of nurses in general), for this effort, and after the 'generous' pay rises announced in April 1988, receives a princely wage of just over £4,800 a year, rising to just under £5,600 by the time she's finished (Londoners get around £1,000 weighting allowance).

In other words a first-level nurse in training is paid at the minimum going rate for a char.

At the end of the course there are examinations, and if she passes (three tries are allowed) the student becomes a staff nurse on a salary scale of £8,025–9,200. (Again, 10 per cent-plus more if she works in inner London.)

Enrolled nurses are an accident of history. When World War II broke out it became necessary to organise an instant increase in the number of hospital beds available in order to be prepared for the handling of an unknown but possibly enormous number of military and civilian casualties. This was largely accomplished by turning some of the huge institutions for the care of the mentally ill and handicapped into general hospitals, and by throwing up a lot of new wards, operating theatres, X-ray departments and so on of a Nissen hut kind in the grounds of these and many small local hospitals.

The new beds had to be staffed – you couldn't suddenly expand the training schools and suddenly find additional thousands of sufficiently educated young women fitted and willing to undergo a rigorous and structured three-year apprenticeship. So the enrolled nurse was born.

Suitable (and doubtless a lot of unsuitable) girls were employed, regardless of their academic prowess, and put on the wards, where they learnt their craft 'on the job', which is the ultimate way anyone really gets to grips with learning how to practise any trade or profession anyway.

After the War was over these emergency nurses began to demand some kind of professional status and job security, and they got what they wanted. The existing wartime recruits were put on a register of state enrolled nurses by virtue of experience, and their caste was enshrined in the nursing scheme of things. New entrants to the grade were (and are) expected to 'provide evidence of having attained a good standard of general education extending over a period of at least ten years'. This delightfully vague requirement made it possible for countless thousands of girls to enter the profession who would earlier have been debarred.

The second-level course usually lasts two years, and involves less (and somewhat less demanding) theoretical work, but just as much devoted labour on the wards. However, an EN can't advance beyond the rank of staff nurse, however meritorious her service or however many post-qualification certificates she obtains. Many excellent second-level nurses, who find themselves performing as well as or better than some of their first-level colleagues, therefore become resentful and frustrated, and feel themselves to be in a dead-end job.

In theory an EN who has shown herself competent *can* become an RN by undergoing a one-year conversion course, which is largely devoted to providing the extra theoretical training contained in the RN curriculum. However, these courses cost hospitals a lot of money, not only because of the teaching facilities and staff needed to run them, but also because the students must still be paid a salary, even though temporarily absent from the regular labour force, where they have to be replaced at yet more expense. Since all hospitals are now desperately short of cash, conversion courses are extremely thin on the ground, and many ENs spend much time and effort writing round the country in usually vain attempts to secure one of the deplorably few conversion-course places available.

At the opposite pole of the class system is the graduate nurse. Graduate nurses are the rule in North America, but here they form a small elite. Nine British universities and polytechnics offer degrees in nursing, and the course lasts four years – a year longer than the normal undergraduate course. This is because, in addition to achieving an academic standard equivalent to that required for any other kind of first degree, the undergraduate nurse must pack in as much practical experience as an RN receives during training.

Nurse undergraduates are paid an ordinary student grant, which varies with the wealth of their parents – just like any other undergraduate. Their fees are paid, however rich their families, and on top of that they receive a maintenance grant which, for the session 1988/89, can be anything from £2,050 (£2,425 in London) to nothing. That's for a 30–week academic year. Undergraduate nurses are required to spend some weeks of their 'vacations' on the wards, and for each of these extra weeks of learning they are paid £42.90 (£55.05 in London), apparently on the strange assumption that fish and chips and rents and newspapers and other staffs of life cost much less during university vacations than at other times. (It's all to do, of course, with some bureaucratic assumption that a pretty large percentage of the maintenance grant is spent on books, and so on, so that extra weeks in harness don't involve a proportional extra expense.)

This may be logical, but it isn't practical. Apart from all else, by the time nurse undergraduates have finished their 'holiday' stints, they find that all the 'holiday' jobs have gone, and they therefore face four years of penury even more wearisome than that suffered by their RN and EN student colleagues.

Once qualified they become staff nurses on an equal footing with RNs, and get no more pay or seniority to compensate them for their extra effort. However, they are perhaps more likely to be in line for fast promotion and appointment to a managerial post.

Midwives usually gain their colours by undergoing an 18-month course at some time after a general training. However, two British schools currently offer a three-year course permitting direct entry to the midwives register, and the comparatively few non-nurse midwives tend to be fiercely proud of their special status. Although many nurses train as midwives, to round off their education, so to speak, and without any intention of devoting their lives to the craft, those who *do* practise regard themselves as independent experts, and by no means simply as aides to the obstetricians. There is currently a strong and growing call for midwives to be allowed to assume full responsibility for the management of the majority of normal pregnancies and labours.

Some 40 institutions of advanced or higher education provide a variety of post-registration courses in fields such as community nursing, occupational health, management and teaching. And within the hospital nurses can qualify as specialists in many branches of clinical medicine and surgery, including intensive care, diseases of the nervous system, paediatrics, cardiology, kidney diseases, orthopaedics, and so on. (A shortage of such specialists has been the primary cause of the postponed heart operations on children which gained so much publicity in 1987 and 1988.)

Other courses for the qualified include one leading to the diploma in nursing. This involves three years of day-release study of an academic kind, during which the emphasis is on the objectives and theory of the art. Needless to say, and as with graduates, those who have gained such a diploma earn no extra pay or recognition, although at the time of writing the government is actively considering ways of encouraging and rewarding those who acquire badly needed special skills.

Nursing auxiliaries are not regarded as nurses at all within the profession, but they certainly are so regarded by the patients they serve. They undertake the mundane tasks like bed-making, bathing and feeding those who require such help, checking temperatures, pulses and respirations, tidying up, and generally serving the simpler, but none the less important, needs of the sick. They will often establish a more intimate relationship with the customer, and provide more immediate comfort and support, than do some of their more skilled colleagues. You don't need any specific qualifications to become an auxiliary, and you learn how to do the job by doing it.

PROBLEMS

Nobody who today opens a newspaper or turns on the radio or television can be unaware of the present discontent within the nursing trade. Poor Florence Nightingale must be shedding hot tears of sadness and despair as she sits in her matron's office in that great hospital in the sky. Her young ladies mounting vulgar demonstrations, waving banners, *and actually going on strike*! Disgraceful! Heartrending! Unthinkable!

Or more likely, she is sitting stern-faced at her desk, busily penning scathing memos to the Lord, outlining the folly and myopia of the bureaucrats and politicians who have allowed such turmoil to develop, and telling Him what to do about it all.

We shall return to these troubles in the final chapter, since the causes of and possible remedies for the current disarray are central to a consideration of the future of the profession which is there discussed. But a brief reminder of what makes nurses mad may be useful now.

Pay, perhaps, is the most obvious and oft-quoted subject of complaint. The Health Department, which is hardly likely to exaggerate such matters, has recently estimated that around 3,000 working nurses are having to claim a family income supplement. This may not seem many out of a labour force of well over half a million, although it is disgraceful that *any* woman providing such a valuable service should find herself classed amongst the indigent. Far more depressing is the department's grim statement that four out of ten nurses are living at poverty level, which presumably means that they have to scrimp and save, and perhaps eat less well than is good for them, and can rarely replace old clothes, whilst still not being quite destitute enough to qualify for a handout from this prosperous 'welfare' state.

However, nobody goes into nursing for the money, and I have gained the strong impression that many nurses might stoically accept the restrictions on their private activities and indulgences imposed by poor pay if it wasn't for the enraging comparison between their own monetary rewards and those enjoyed by, say, firemen and the police. The size of their pay packets makes them feel devalued by society.

Nurses *do* go into nursing because of a strong desire to care for people, and much of their present frustration arises from an inability to do the job as well as they feel it should and could be done.

There is a shortage of nurses, partly due to a shortage of cash, and this means that those who remain have too much to do. There is not enough time to give individual patients the attention they should have, and junior nurses are often left to shoulder responsibilities beyond their courage and experience.

A lot can't stand the pressure, and leave, which just makes things worse for those who remain. Of all the nurses in training, almost a quarter will drop out before qualifying, and around 1,000 of the 20,000 or so who do qualify each year then stop work. Increasing numbers of qualified NHS staff, and particularly those with special skills, are moving to jobs abroad or in the private sector, where they find better means for doing the job, and not just better pay.

The shortage (and therefore the pressures) seems set to increase unless some pretty radical steps are taken to make the profession much more attractive to school leavers. By the early 1990s, because of a falling birth rate in the 1970s, the number of girls leaving school with the qualifications needed for entry to the profession will have fallen by a quarter. Thus, even if the same proportion of eligible young ladies choose nursing as a career, the shortfall of recruits will be disastrous. Added to this, though, banks, department stores, public relations firms, and a host of other service industries, are creating more and more jobs for bright school leavers which are far less demanding, as well as offering more cash.

A high proportion of nurses, particularly among the more junior ranks, 'moonlight' in order to make ends meet. The country is studded with agencies which supply nurse 'temps' to short-staffed NHS hospitals as well as private institutions. The agencies charge rates well in excess of the wages earned by regular staff, although the girls they employ get only marginally more than they would for the same hours of work in their own establishments (except that NHS nurses get more than their normal hourly reward when farmed out to the private sector).

Moonlighting keeps many nurses solvent, but often at the cost of exhaustion when it occupies time which should be spent sleeping or just unwinding from an already gruelling routine. It's one extra stress, perhaps self-imposed, but imposed out of necessity and certainly not because of greed.

The nurses I've spoken to are clearly proud of their profession and love their work. Those who are wondering whether they should pack it in contemplate the possibility with regret, and only at all because they cannot see how, if they stay, they can ever hope to own a car, or a home of their own, or many of the other rewards of hard and skilled work which the rest of us take for granted.

CHANGES

In the good old days the nursing hierarchy was relatively simple. You had probationers, staff nurses, sisters (called charge nurses when male), matrons and assistant matrons, and everybody knew where they were. But since the war successive governments have vainly hoped that the many and growing problems attached to maintaining a complex and enormous structure of medical care (the NHS is far and away the largest employer in the land) could somehow be coralled and controlled by undertaking various kinds of 'reorganisation' of the bureaucracy running the affair. Often these 'reorganisations' have been based on the recommendations of some academic or business tycoon with no hands-on experience of caring for the sick, and they have usually involved giving the same old bunch of executives and committee-men a new set of titles and notional responsibilities. One result of all this tinkering has been that there is now a bewildering array of nursing grades, with most of the new ones having an administrative role.

As a consequence (and this is a cause of widespread complaint) a nurse can only achieve promotion beyond a certain level, and therefore earn a half-respectable wage, by forsaking the bedside and going into management. This may suit some (and especially, it seems, the men), but most nurses go into nursing because they want to nurse – to care for patients. So there is currently a demand that the career structure should be modified so that good and experienced practical clinicians can spend a professional lifetime working at the sharp end without sacrificing the higher status and pay which ability and seniority should attract.

Another recent gimmick has been to import 'managers' from outside the NHS, such as ex-soldiers and businessmen, in a bid to 'increase efficiency', which is the term our present lords and mistresses at Westminster use when they mean 'cut costs'. Some of the immigrants have fitted in well enough, but many have met, and have perhaps invited, hostility. Anyway, and rightly or wrongly, a lot of nurses are inclined to blame a high proportion of their present difficulties on the fact that their affairs are under the control of people who wouldn't know a bedpan from a tourniquet. Nursing, say nurses, should be run by nurses.

However, the changes which have occurred so far are as nothing compared to those proposed. The present Conservative government is clearly determined to change the shape and nature of the NHS, and has the time and clout to have its way, whatever the labourers in the vineyard and their customers may feel about the wisdom of disrupting a system which, despite shortcomings, provides a generally excellent service of health care more economically than any yet devised elsewhere.

The main aim would appear to be to change the financing of medicine so that far more of the cost is met by the consumer, either through insurance or some other means, rather than by general taxation. A corollary is that the users would have greater choice – that doctors and hospitals would have to compete for customers – and that many citizens, perhaps a majority, would turn to the private sector for most of their medical needs.

Whatever the outcome of the current scheming and debates, the pattern of nursing is bound to be affected. Some nurses might even find themselves properly paid if their services had to be purchased in the market-place. Whether they would find a new system provided them with better opportunities for doing a proper job of work is altogether a different matter.

But meanwhile the UKCC is proposing a radical revamp of the profession along lines described in a plan which the council has christened Project 2000, after the year in which, with a bit of luck, the dreams it incorporates may have come true. This, too, we shall look at in more detail in the final chapter.

The main thrust of Project 2000 (which owes nothing to any political ideologies) is to upgrade the status of British nurses, and to start by tackling the training course. At the moment student nurses spend much of their time on the wards and in other hospital departments, where they form a significant element of the labour force. They are landed with many of the more tedious chores, like emptying bedpans and turning patients to prevent the development of bedsores, with the worst jobs going to the most junior, and the more glamorous tasks like renewing dressings or helping with medicine rounds or escorting patients to the operating theatre being the preserve of the more senior girls. Often enough a student finds herself left in charge, especially at night when there's a shortage of hands or when the staff nurse on duty has gone for her meal break. There's usually help at hand, 'somewhere down the corridor', but at times these sessions in the driving seat can be quite frightening.

So, and with ample justification, students feel themselves regarded as a pool of cheap labour, and complain that they are not so much being taught as being used.

The UKCC aims to change all that. It wants nurses in training to be treated as proper students. Their three-year course will have a high and broad academic content, and although they will still be given ample practical experience, both within hospitals and in other settings, they will always be supernumeraries, and will not be counted or depended upon as impressed workhorses. They will end up (and, it is hoped, be regarded) more like graduates than humble apprentices who have served their time.

But there's a snag. Since they won't (in theory, at least) be doing any work for the NHS, they won't receive the rich cash reward at present earned by a student nurse. Just like nursing undergraduates, they'll have to make do on the equivalent of a student grant.

And there's another snag. The proposed course will be the common and only port of entry to the profession, and the two-level system will disappear. All nurses will thereafter belong to the 'officer class'; the squaddies and NCOs will be the nursing auxiliaries, or whatever new subordinate ranks are invented, and they won't be counted as nurses at all. So what's going to happen to the SENs?

Well, that's what *they* want to know. Project 2000 contains the proposal that the further recruitment and training of enrolled nurses should cease quite soon, but also insists that ample provision should be made for enabling 'suitable' existing SENs to show themselves worthy of promotion to the officers' mess. In view of the miserably inadequate availability of conversion courses within the present regime, not many SENs believe that such pious statements of intent are likely to result in any substantial improvement of their prospects. SENs are therefore now a particularly bolshie and discontented section of the nursing trade.

And a lot of others concerned for the survival of an excellent system of health care wonder where the 20,000–odd new nurses

needed every year are to come from if boys and girls who don't
cope very well with maths and French and geography at school are
to be considered unsuited to the task.

You don't have to be a good scholar to be a good nurse.

You just have to be intelligent, industrious, compassionate –
and tough.

Chapter 2

A GRADUATE NURSE

Marie-Louise Curtin is a nursing graduate and, at the age of 27, a junior sister at Atkinson Morley's Hospital in southwest London. This is one of the world's leading centres for the treatment of diseases and injuries affecting the nervous system. Sister Curtin began her undergraduate course in 1978 at Chelsea College (now incorporated with King's College) in the University of London.

My mother was a trained midwife and a district nurse, so right from the word go I had a good idea of what the job entails, how difficult it is, and the stamina it demands.

I was head-girl of my school, and with 13 O-levels and three good A-levels in German, French and history I had quite a wide choice of career. I wanted to go to university, and would really have liked to study modern languages, but couldn't see how that would lead to any job I'd enjoy.

Then I discovered you could do a degree in nursing, so I thought 'I'll go for that.' I'd have a qualification, and could always *not* be a nurse at the end of it, and could go on and do, say, linguistics.

So that was my basic motivation – not a desire to care for people.

The degree course was a very traumatic and schizophrenic business. On the one hand we were students, living in a students'

16

residence, belonging to the union, and doing all the studenty things, and on the other hand we were nurses. We'd attend lectures at the university, which were excellent, and then have to change into uniform and become a student nurse; there was a great chasm between the two lifestyles. We did the practical work at the Charing Cross, which is a particularly fine hospital.

I liked the relationship between lecturers and students at the college, but I *didn't* like the didactic way the student nurses were being taught.

And because we had practical nursing experience spread right through the course there were some evenings when you couldn't stay all night at a party, for example, because you had to turn up for early duty next day.

We were aware of a general atmosphere within the hospital – a feeling among some of the nurses that we were high-flying intellectual pseudo-nurses, and that we'd just get our degree and then fly off into administration. That was a cliché I'll never forget. Actually a higher proportion of graduates than RGNs *stay* in the clinical field.

At college we were taught how things *should* be done. We learned an idealistic way of nursing, and the philosophies involved, which are actually quite complicated and have been very well thought out – mostly by Americans. And then we went on the wards, and, of course, ideals never match reality. We'd say 'Why can't we change this?' and 'Why can't you do it like that?' and this may have caused a bit of friction, and there *were* some prejudices. But it's a matter of personality, really, and how well you can get on and mix.

So it could be very traumatic and difficult. There were 25 of us on the course to start with, and 18 at the finish, but that's about the same drop-out rate that you find in any nursing school. Quite a high proportion of the survivors of my group are now sisters, and some have gone into research.

But despite the tribulations I thoroughly enjoyed the course, and I think I derived a lot of experience and advantage from the contrast between college and hospital in the end, because it did teach us to be very flexible and adaptable. And at college we had seminars, and experience of giving talks and presenting arguments, which helps when it comes to talking to registrars and quite senior doctors.

By the time I graduated I knew I wanted to be a nurse.

FIRST JOB

Because I wanted some management experience and to learn, as a staff nurse, how to run a ward, I joined a very progressive geriatric intensive care unit. That's not intensive care of a technical kind, but intensive care in the literal sense of the word. We dealt with very old people who had basically *crumbled* at home, for whatever reason. And we set out to rehabilitate them, and get them back into the community, rather than have them eke out an existence in a long-stay ward.

I know people wrinkle their noses when they hear the word 'geriatrics', because it's still regarded as a low-status specialty, but I loved it – absolutely loved it.

I think one of the most valuable skills I learnt there was how to manage people. If you can persuade an old lady who really knows her own mind, particularly if she doesn't want to *do* anything – 'I'm quite happy here, thank you very much', and she doesn't really want to go home, even though she knows it would be much better for her – if you can motivate somebody like that to get up and to use her walking-frame properly, and to *take* her tablets, and you can persuade her to look after herself, and she *does*, and she goes out, and is happier – that's brilliant. It's a matter of discovering how to organise people, and how to talk to them on a very *sensible* level. How not to be patronising. How not to be dominant because you're the one in uniform. There's a very well-ordered body language between nurse and patient – 'I'm the nurse, I'm in uniform, I know what I'm talking about, and *you* do it. *You* have no say.' That's changing, because we're encouraging people to participate in their own care. If people understand what you're trying to do they *will* cooperate, because they know it's for their own good. So there's a lot of psychology and psychosocial relationship involved.

Our turnover was quite fast, and in order to be successful I had to develop my coordination skills. We had to liaise with the physiotherapists, the occupational therapists, the social work-ers, the housing people, the community nurses, the community physicians, the physicians in the hospital, the dieticians. In a nutshell you çan say a large part of the nurse's time and skills are spent on being a very good coordinator of all the avail-able resources.

On that unit it was the nurses who had the closest contact with the patients. The doctors were there mainly to do ward rounds, and very often whether the patients did well or not depended on how good the nurses were.

SURGERY

After that I became a senior staff nurse on an extremely acute surgical ward.

That was a different kettle of fish altogether because we were dealing with quite major stuff. One half of the ward was given over to vascular surgery – repair of aortic aneurysms, bypass grafts, that sort of thing. The other half was for patients undergoing gastrointestinal surgery, and some of that was quite amazing. There were drips and drains hanging out everywhere, and some patients were being fed entirely through intravenous tubes. It was the sort of ward where anything could happen. Somebody would have a cardiac arrest, and then there'd be another, or somebody would start to bleed. That was when I really came into contact with the nursing process and how to plan *individual* care for patients.

Nursing used to be mostly task-orientated. There would be one nurse to do the washing, and another to do all the observations, and another to do all the dressings. You'd take turns. That was good for reducing stress levels, because it's much more stressful to be responsible for the *total* care of four or six patients. But even though it's more stressful, it's much better, both for the nurse and the patient, if you've got *one* person looking after those four or six people. They *know* who their nurse is. There's rapport and trust and confidence built up. And that's very important in treating people, because you won't get cooperation and really good results without it.

I think I enjoyed the surgery most. I loved the geriatrics, but for different reasons.

ATKINSON MORLEY'S

At this point I'd been qualified for two-and-a-half years, and I had to decide what to do next.

On some of my days off I'd done agency work. Because of our financial situation nurses very often do agency work, just to earn a few extra pounds. So I did some work on the neurosurgical unit at the Royal Free and found myself absolutely fascinated by what was going on. I decided I'd like to do another course and specialise in the subject.

Atkinson Morley's has a very good reputation, so I came here to work as a staff nurse for six months to discover whether that was what I really wanted to do. I found it was, and I did the neurosciences course. It's a six-month course which is run by quite a few neuro centres in this country – very intensive, jam packed with a *lot* of knowledge, very complex, very interesting, and very challenging. The lectures are integrated with clinical teaching, and we worked all round the hospital, taking in all the different specialities, including rehabilitation, intensive care, neurosurgery, neurology, and neuropaediatrics. You end up with the certificate in neurosurgical and neuromedical nursing.

I carried on working here afterwards as a senior staff nurse, and then a junior sister's post came up, which is what I am now.

I'm working on a female neurosurgical ward, dealing with people who've had traumatic bleeds – subarachnoid haemorrhages and intracerebral bleeds – and people with various tumours of the brain and spinal cord, or infarctions, or back problems. Anything, really, to do with the nervous system.

We can do things as simple as a carpal-tunnel release, but we do extremely major surgery as well. It's very acute stuff, and you do need highly specialised knowledge to look after people well. You have to be very well trained in the skill of observing the patient, and knowing the nervous signs that occur when somebody's deteriorating, which are not so obvious, perhaps, as they might be in other kinds of illness. You have to understand what's happening in the brain, and that knowledge allows you to anticipate what might come next and to do something to stop it – to treat people with life-threatening problems and prevent them from dying.

There's an added strain on my ward because of the age range. At the moment we have an 11-year-old girl who's had a massive intracerebral bleed – *11 years old*! And you have young men of 22 who are dying of brain tumours. You're dealing with awfully distressed relatives, and it takes all your energy and determination to handle the situation properly. And knowing that if you *miss* something – you don't recognise that a patient's deteriorating very slowly and you don't call a doctor – somebody could be very badly damaged.

But very often I find that *my* knowledge – because I've done the course and worked in the field for two-and-a-half years – is better than that of a senior house officer who's new to the job. Non-medical people always assume that the doctor knows better than the nurse.

Staff shortages don't make life any easier. In my own ward we're only using *nine* beds out of 22, and the paediatric ward is having to take some women mixed in with the children.

Not so many people are going into nursing, for obvious reasons, and they're dropping out faster. Women who've left to have families aren't coming back, and others are going abroad. You can earn £22,000 as a staff nurse in California, so if you've nothing to keep you here, why not have a go?

We had to stop admitting patients for a time last summer, so somebody smashed up outside and needing acute neurosurgery would have had to be taken to Southampton, by which time he might have died, and it very nearly happened. So that was upsetting, but we just didn't have the nurses, and for those of us who were left the pressure was unbelievable.

It's hard finding yourself in charge of a shift made up entirely of agency nurses you've never met before. They'll all be qualified, but that doesn't mean anything. You may have ten patients who are very sick and in need of a lot of attention. How do you dole them out when you don't know how competent the individual nurses are?

It's all very rewarding – but it's *very* stressful.

HOW ARE WE DOING?

Nursing is becoming much more of a research-based profession. We have to be accountable for what we do, and to record what we do very accurately. If you can't write it down, and if you can't actually demonstrate on paper what you've done and show how the patient benefited, that's really a major failing.

People have been looking into the things nurses *have* been doing and saying 'Yes, we've shown that's very good and very beneficial' or 'We've shown this does no good whatsoever, so why are people doing it still?'

We've been using a modified American system called Monitor which is based on observations and keeping a score, which should make it possible to assess the standard of nursing care, which you can then use to compare wards within hospitals, or hospital with hospital. A team of outside assessors comes round and they observe certain things and ask the patients certain questions: 'Did the nurse introduce herself to you?' 'Did she show you where the toilets were?' 'Did she tell you when the next meal was coming?' 'Did she tell you about the services available?' 'Did she give you a booklet?' 'Does the nurse always come when you call?' 'Do you feel unsafe?' They are *personal* things, reflecting how the patients feel the nurses are dealing with them, and they record a 'Yes', 'No', or 'Not applicable' answer. Then they'll talk to the nurses: 'How often do you change the intravenous giving set?' 'What are you cleaning this wound with?' 'When was that dressing last changed?' 'Do you know about the condition of this patient?' 'What's the diagnosis?'

These are just examples. There are over 160 very wide-ranging questions, and it takes a number of days to assess a ward. Then they'll go away and add it all up and make recommendations. Ideally, they'll come back six months or a year later and do it all over again, so if you've notched up a poor score you do have an opportunity to improve. It's happening all over the country, and there's a special course to train assessors.

This may all sound very 'finger-pointing', and it could be seen as threatening, but I think it's healthy, and people shouldn't be afraid. And it can be very useful to be able to say 'Look, Monitor says this is really not acceptable any more, so please Mr General Manager can we have some more money?'

PROJECT 2000

I agree with the philosophy and principles behind the scheme – striving to raise the status of nurses and making nursing more of a recognised profession. And one way of doing that, it is *thought*, is to create an academically highly-qualified corps.

But there's a conflict of needs. Because of the nursing shortage it's very difficult to see how you can keep thousands of students out of the labour force and in a college for some long time, although I'd very much like to see that happen. And nursing is *not* about having the highest qualifications in the land. You can have three A-levels, but be absolutely socially inept and have no communication skills and have *no* common sense, which means you wouldn't do very well as a nurse.

You'll find really good, sensible, practical, enrolled nurses running wards. They don't have the same qualifications as RGNs, and therefore they shouldn't have the same responsibilities or be subjected to the same stresses, but they are. They're not getting paid the same as an RGN who's doing the same job, and they have nowhere to *go*. They can't become sisters.

A lot of girls only become enrolled nurses because they were ill-informed at school, which is awful. They could very well have qualified for RGN training, but nobody *told* them. I don't know whether it's poor career advisers or poor publicity by nursing itself. I'd like to see a good mix of opportunities for entering the profession.

There's a real role for male nurses. Often they don't come straight from school. They've done other degrees or jobs, and have then suddenly decided, for some reason, that they'd like to do nursing. And that gives them certain qualities which ordinary school-leavers don't have. A lot of top nurses and top nursing managers are men.

MONEY

The money angle's a sore point.

At the moment I'm a fairly financially independent single woman living in a staff flat, but there's no way I could think of buying a flat for myself.

My basic salary is £9,000, I've been nursing for nine years, my unsocial hours are absolutely horrendous, and I have the pressure of running a very acute ward. If I wanted to buy a flat and pay out a rather heavy mortgage – if I *had* to afford it somehow – then I'd have to leave nursing and go into something else offering better pay.

Having said that, I'm not sure I ever would.

I'm very optimistic that eventually we'll get something, because scarce commodities become extremely valuable, and nurses are becoming very scarce. We ought to be remunerated for any extra courses we undertake. And there's a huge gap between the London weighting given to nurses and policemen, for example, which is very strange.

THE CUSTOMERS

Most people coming into hospital, unless they've got a problem that makes them confused and disorientated so that you can't have a sensible conversation, say 'Oh, I didn't realise you worked so hard, I didn't realise you were *so* short-staffed, I didn't realise you had to cope with all this busy-ness and turnover and stress.'

And then they say 'I really think you ought to be paid more.'

And I say 'Who's your local MP? You ought to write to him.'

And they say 'Oh well...'

'I'll give you a stamped addressed envelope.'

And then they go away and think 'It's a really nice hospital. It was *really* good.' And they forget about it.

I wouldn't like to count on any active support from the customers. Nurses are angels one minute, but if ever we went on strike, or could be seen to damage any area of health care, it would be a different story.

And I don't think you'd ever find a nurse who hasn't been subjected to abuse and assault. It happens a lot in accident and emergency departments, for obvious reasons, with people coming in drunk, or who don't want to be brought in at all. And you have angry and distressed relatives. Verbal abuse is commonest, but I've been the butt of physical violence at least once.

You must always try to remember that this person doesn't hate you personally. They don't *know* you. It's because they're suffering such terrific stress and anxiety themselves, so they release it in aggression. They have to take it out on *somebody*. And because you're there in uniform, and seen to be controlling things, they take it out on you.

I'd never ever, ever lose my temper with somebody, even if they're really horrible. And some of them have been *really* horrible. When they calm down they're usually terribly apologetic.

I say 'Don't worry about it – I realise.'

DOCTORS

I get on with doctors very well on the whole. It's amazing how, as your uniform changes, as you become more senior, the quality of contact changes.

If *I* think they're wrong I certainly tell them, but I always back up anything I say with very good reasons. If they give *me* good reasons for thinking such-and-such when I've raised a query, and they're not just being arrogant, and they can justify what they say, then all right, fair enough.

You often hear the complaint that nurses are treated as doctors' handmaidens, but when that happens it's because a nurse has *allowed* herself to be treated like that. I think a lot of the blame lies at the nurse's door, because we *are* clinical practitioners, and we are professionals in our own right. Our training is different, but it is not any *less* than a doctor's. Perhaps he knows more about a lot of things – I couldn't do an operation – but equally *he* couldn't do a lot of things that I know very well.

If you've got a sensible chap he'll realise pretty soon that he's got a good team of nurses working for him. And I *do* like doctors who take an interest in the nursing *side* of things, and don't just disappear off the ward round without asking what you've been doing for a patient – what the skin condition's like, whether you've been feeding her.

Basically there's a good integration and exchange of ideas between doctors and nurses, and nurses are now getting accustomed to being quite vocal and standing up for themselves. There *are* the very traditional consultants who are extremely irrational and unreasonable and who become angry for no good cause. They tend to be the older ones. Having said that, I've just thought of one consultant who wasn't particularly old, and who was absolutely arrogant, and probably the worst of the lot, and I can think of many older consultants who are really *very* nice. Maybe it depends on what sort of experience they've had with nurses in the past, and sometimes their politeness varies with the seniority of the nurse being spoken to.

And sometimes I see patients being not very well spoken to. There's poor communication. '*I'm* a doctor, I'm telling you this, *you* will listen, *don't* ask questions.'

DEATH

Everybody has their own individual way of coping. Very often I think it depends on your past experience of death within your own personal background. Deaths do tend to make me terribly sad. When you nurse somebody you get to know them quite well, and you get to know the family. Coping with young people dying is much more difficult. When an old person dies it's more acceptable.

The support of colleagues is extremely important. If you have a good team round you, you tend to find that the sorrow and pressures are spread. I think a lot of nurses share these things and talk them out.

PROSPECTS

At this moment in my career I'm extremely happy. I've got my
junior sister's post. We're making great moves on the ward. We've
got a good atmosphere going. We've recruited five more nurses,
which will make a *big* difference. So morale is quite high. And
my personal life is very happy as well. One tends to affect the
other quite a lot. So at the moment I can foresee myself nursing
for quite a few years to come.

I can carry on in the neurosciences and possibly become a senior
sister, or possibly go into a senior nurse post, although that's much
more concerned with management, which doesn't appeal to me
just now as I wouldn't have a ward.

I could go back into general surgery and perhaps become a
clinical nurse manager, retaining some footing in the clinical field
as an adviser and clinical specialist.

I could go into any other branch of nursing based on the ward.
I could go into research to look at some basic problems and try
to improve the way nurses operate. There's quite a lot of money
around for nursing research and it's just a matter of getting to
know which funds are available.

I could take a two-year course to become a nurse tutor, or study
to become a lecturer and teach degree nursing in a university. Or
I could go into the community after doing a course in district
nursing, or health visiting, or midwifery. There's a wide variety
of things I could do if I really wanted a change.

Not many of my non-medical friends could say that they always
enjoy going to work, but I actually do. When I come back from
holiday I sit here and think 'Oh, I wonder who's on today' and
'I wonder what happened to Mrs So-and-so.'

If I don't have quite a few laughs at work – laugh with the
patients, have quite a relaxed time – I think there's something very
wrong. Other people who work in offices find it boring and they
hate it. They may be very highly paid, but it's very unfulfilling for
them. In nursing you get back what you put in, and far more as
well. So it's very rewarding, but it's a very hard, demanding job,
both mentally and physically, especially with night duty thrown
in. And I have found that friends who've left nursing for more

highly-paid jobs with better hours often look so much fitter and less tired than they used to as nurses.

Despite all that, and knowing what I know now, I think I'd start all over again, simply because I find it very hard to think of another job in which whatever talents I have could be utilised quite so well.

Chapter 3

ENROLLED NURSE

Marian Sharpe is an enrolled nurse, aged 24, who qualified five years ago after two years' training at St Bartholomew's Hospital. She is just ending a one-year course at the Hospital for Sick Children (commonly known as Great Ormond Street or GOS) leading to a certificate in paediatric cardiothoracic intensive care. She lives in her own modern and pleasant flat in Putney, which she shares with a friend, and has a mortgage to repay.

I love babies. I absolutely adore children.

I joined the St John Ambulance Brigade when I was 13. The lady in charge was the sister running the paediatric unit at the local hospital, so I did a lot of voluntary work there. I used to put on uniform and go there after school and at weekends, and I really enjoyed that. You'd get another stripe on your uniform for every 1,000 hours you did. I also went to a home for disabled ex-servicemen. I used to talk to them and write letters for them.

I didn't spend much time on schoolwork because I was more interested in my voluntary work, so I only got O-levels in human biology and needlework and cookery – the rest were just CSEs.

I left school at 16 and went to college, but gave up and went to London as a nanny, working with children again, and I had full charge of a baby and a toddler. Then I was offered a place at Bart's to do the SEN training.

BART'S

I started at Bart's in 1981, and I absolutely *adored* my training. I loved every single minute of it.

It's a very old-fashioned hospital. They're quite strict and have rules and regulations, and that's what I enjoyed. And I think that's what nursing lacks now. People just don't care what they do and what they wear and what they look like.

They were very careful not to segregate the SEN and SRN students. We wore the same uniforms and the same navy-blue belts, but as soon as we qualified they took the blue belts away and gave us green belts instead. And yet we were expected to do exactly the same amount of work and take exactly the same amount of responsibility. Nobody has ever turned round to me and said 'You can't do *that* – you're only an SEN.' I've taken charge of wards when there have been SRNs there as well, but who just couldn't do it. I was once left in charge of the cardiac unit when I'd just got into my second year. I was 19 years old. At the time I thought 'Oh, great! I know exactly what I'm doing.' But looking back, and after my last year's experience in intensive care, I've wondered how I could have coped if something had gone wrong. And things *did* go wrong, but no-one took much notice. They just *used* us. But Bart's does have very high standards, and I don't know how SENs would compare with SRNs in other schools round the country.

We did get a lot of support when we were students, perhaps more so because the wards were the old-fashioned Nightingale type. They weren't split up into cubicles and odd spaces round corners, so you could always see sister on the unit. She was never in her office, which was quite a long way off the ward: she'd always be sat at her desk. And you could always see your staff nurse. So if there was ever a problem they were with you straightaway.

So we did have a lot of support. Not so much in the way of teaching, but the staff were actually sharing the work; they were rolling up their sleeves in the morning and getting on with it. If there were three of us, and 25 blanket baths to do, they'd be doing half. I think staff nurses these days feel they don't have to do any of the chores, that they're there to do the book-keeping and paperwork and go walking around with the doctors. That's not good enough.

As soon as I qualified I went to work in the paediatric unit, which is a 20–bed general ward, and it's extremely busy. We used to get anything and everything in. I stayed there for three-and-a-half years. But even then, when I was on the staff, *I'd* get my sleeves up. I'd do baby baths. I always said 'Don't leave all the dirty work to the students.' Every day I always made sure I did something that nobody else wanted to do. If the students saw that *we* were doing something dirty, they didn't mind cleaning the sluice up themselves. No-one likes the nasty jobs, but why leave it all to the students? It's important to keep your relationships right with your students. If you treat them fairly they'll work well for you.

There were 16 in our set when I started in '81. I actually live with one of the girls now. She gave up nursing just before her finals – she'd had enough, she couldn't take any more. And others went for various reasons. I think there are three of us now who are still in nursing. They liked their training, but a lot of girls got pregnant. We lived in the nurses' home, in extremely small rooms, and with no chance of getting anywhere else. We were living in the City at the time, and they left to have babies just to get themselves rehoused – they got flats in the Barbican. It does still happen, but less and less, because they're being put into bed-and-breakfast now for a time, instead of straight into nice accommodation. Six or seven girls from my set left for that reason.

While I was on the children's ward I began to feel the time had come to do my conversion course. Bart's weren't running one, because they hadn't the money to spare, and I began writing endless letters to other hospitals and getting replies saying 'No course available' or 'We only want nurses from our own area health authority'. So I thought the next best thing was to go off and qualify for a post-registration certificate, which would show that I could study, and give me a better chance of being accepted for conversion.

GREAT ORMOND STREET

Since I'd spent so long on the children's ward, I applied to GOS. They told me not to do straight paediatrics, but to do the cardiothoracic intensive care course because it's a lot more interesting. But I haven't enjoyed the last year.

At the moment we don't have enough work to do because we haven't sufficient staff to do many operations. Sometimes they have the ward staff but don't have the theatre staff, or then they get the theatre staff but the ward staff have left. It's a vicious circle, and less and less work gets done.

We work 13–hour shifts, three days a week, and it's soul-destroying going in and knowing you're there for 13 hours with not enough to do, unless an emergency comes in. You can't get on with the job. You're forever taking patients to the theatre, and as soon as you get to the anaesthetic room the operation's cancelled – sometimes for the third, fourth or fifth time. The patients have had their pre-med, but you have to take them back to the ward. The parents are there, all teed-up for their child having to undergo major heart surgery, and it's my job to explain what's happened. OK, the doctors will come down later, but the parents get very cross with us, and although it's not our fault they take their anxiety and frustration out on us initially.

Or sometimes the surgeons will decide in the afternoon that they can, after all, fit a patient in, but the child's had lunch, so the operation has to be cancelled again. It doesn't make for a very good working atmosphere. We get extremely cross with the doctors, and the parents get furious with *us*.

Another thing – we students have to share the canteen facilities with the parents. So as soon as you get down there and try to relax in this filthy room (no curtains, it's absolutely disgusting, our sitting room in GOS), the parents want to come up to us and ask us questions. You can never get away from them. The doctors have a lovely sitting room with double glazing, curtains, carpets, television, newspapers. They've spent thousands doing that room up for them, yet the student nurses have got nothing. They've got a *nice* sitting room for the trained staff who work there full time, but because we're students we don't get to use it.

The canteen's shut when we want some food. There's no hot food at weekends. You can have sandwiches taken out of the freezer. It's just one thing after another. It sounds petty, but if you're on intensive care, and there's no food in the kitchen – because, obviously, the patients don't eat – you can go all day without eating. The theory is that you can take food in with you. But we work 13 hours a day for three days at a stretch each week, and I don't have *time* to buy the food to take in with me. It does sound rather pathetic. But when you go to work and there's nothing to eat, it's not very enjoyable.

We don't have a proper changing room with lockers, just a filthy kind of toilet. And somebody gets something stolen almost every week. You can't leave your handbag in the office, and I have to carry all my credit cards and cheque book in my uniform, which isn't exactly ideal in intensive care.

But I can't say I've been particularly overworked at GOS. The ratio of nurses to patients is extremely high. They're waiting to go into a new cardiac wing which has been built for the last ten years, but soon after it opened the ceilings started cracking and they had to move back into the old unit while it's being repaired, which meant being restricted to ten beds again. They keep saying all these problems will be solved once they get back into the new wing. Meanwhile they've built the staff up against the day when they'll be needed, so they've got about 20 sisters for a ten-bed paediatric unit.

There's a lot of unrest, because they're promoting everybody, just to stop them leaving, and the sisters who've worked hard to get where they are aren't very pleased to find staff nurses being made sisters after they've been qualified for just six months. I don't like it either. I've been nursing for seven years now, and I've so much experience, yet I can't progress, and I see these girls who've been qualified for six or eight months getting sisters' posts. That's what's upsetting a lot of enrolled nurses. They think 'Why stay? There's just no point. Let's go and do something else.'

The quality of nursing care provided by the staff who are doing the cardiothoracic course is very high, because we're interested in what we're doing, and in getting on, and we've all come from reasonably good training hospitals, but I find some of the staff who've been there a long time couldn't give a damn about the patients. They're only interested in all the hi-tech surgery and the new equipment and monitoring equipment, and the basic nursing care has completely gone out of the window.

I'm very interested in all the machinery, and the reasons why we do this and that, and drug interactions, and technical matters in general, but you mustn't forget that the patients need simple nursing care as well. I've taken children back to the general wards from intensive care with terrible pressure sores on their necks from the ventilator rolls used to keep their necks extended, and their mouths have been filthy, and they've got ulcerations from the ventilator tube round their noses, purely because the staff can't be bothered to look after them properly.

Some of the permanent staff have done the course, and others haven't, but they've been there a long time, and I think they're frightened to leave because they've forgotten most of what they knew, apart from cardiothoracic intensive care. They've got a nice little job, and are quite happy.

I've made a lot of complaints to the school of nursing about it, but nothing has been done. They won't *say* anything to the nurses in case they just turn round and say 'Right! Keep your job! I'll go somewhere else.'

I've worked in the general intensive care unit, and in neonatal intensive care, and the standards there are extremely high. And the standard of the surgery is fantastic. But that's not down to the English doctors. That's due to all the American doctors who've just come over to the unit. This time last year I'd say we were having seven or eight deaths a week, if not more, but since the Americans arrived and there's been a change of staff and they've modified some of the procedures, the rate's dropped considerably, so that now we might be losing one or two or three a week.

I'm afraid I've painted rather a grim picture of GOS. But I haven't enjoyed the last year, and I shall be glad to leave.

MOONLIGHTING

I couldn't possibly afford a flat of my own out of my NHS
pay. My outgoings – mortgage, life assurance, maintenance, rates
– come to nearly £500 a month, not taking into account food and
travelling expenses, and I take home £550, which would leave me
£50 to live on. So I've been working four or five nights a month for
an agency, which sees me through. And if I do another night on
top of that I can go out and buy a new pair of shoes, or a bottle
of perfume, or something.

I feel I've got quite a high standard of living and I'm not
on the bread line, but to get what I've got I sometimes have to
do back-to-back shift work, going all day and all night. And I'm
fortunate enough to have parents who've helped me out quite a
bit with the flat. A lot of girls don't have parents who are in a
position to do that.

The agency I'm with specialises in paediatrics and intensive care,
and they charge private clients a lot more than general agencies
can. If I do a night in the private sector I take home £60, which
is pretty good going, but I quite often opt for a night shift in an
NHS hospital, even though that only pays £40, because I'd rather
be able to look forward to going to work instead of dreading the
prospect. I'd *never* work full-time in the private sector.

Private hospitals are terribly overstaffed. The hours are good,
the facilities are lovely, the food's lovely, and so are the sitting
areas for the nurses. And there's a good working relationship with
the doctors, because they're there for the money just as much as we
are, and they have to treat the nurses well, otherwise we'd leave,
and with no staff they'd have no patients. But nursing foreigners
is *very* demanding.

There's a constant problem of communication. There are not
many interpreters, because they're difficult to get hold of. To work
full-time in the Harley Street Clinic you actually have to learn
Arabic. And you're at the patients' beck and call constantly. If they
say they don't want you in the room, you have to get out, whatever
you may be doing. They think that because they're paying they
own the place. They walk around and do what they like, and have
visitors whenever they want, and in the main they're very rude to

the nurses. They actually *spit* at us. There are one or two clinics I won't work in any more.

I haven't had a whole weekend off for two or three years now, or cooked a Sunday dinner, or enjoyed a good lie-in. I could do with a break from agency work.

AMBITION AND FRUSTRATION

I've done a year's work at GOS. They're desperate for trained cardiothoracic nurses, and they've asked me to stay, but I won't because they've nothing to offer me. They don't do a conversion course because they're only concerned with paediatrics. So I'm going to St Thomas', where they do run a course, and hopefully, if I work hard enough and show that I'm willing and capable, they'll let me on it.

I'll be working in the theatres and the recovery area. We had a good look round when I went for my interview, and everyone was very nice. Sister introduced me to the anaesthetist in charge of the unit, and he said 'The nurses run this unit. They know best. We don't interfere.' I thought 'Oh, great! This sounds quite good.' It seemed a good working atmosphere. There's a nice canteen looking out over the river, and plenty of food – *not* like GOS.

They gave me a long list of dos and don'ts. Your hair's got to be tied up properly, no earrings and no jewelry, no make-up. There were detailed instructions about how to look after their famous spotted muslin cap, how to wash it frequently and hang it upside down over the bath. I think 'OK, that's old-fashioned, but at least they have some standards.' Whereas at GOS nurses wear dozens of earrings, and scruffy uniforms, and have holes in their tights and filthy old shoes. There's no way *I'd* ever go to work like that. If you're talking to parents and talking to doctors you've got to look pretty smart or they wouldn't have any confidence in you. Thomas' has got the reputation for being quite snooty, but the more people tell me that, the happier I am to be going there.

If I get my conversion course I'd stay at Tommy's for at least another two years after that. That's part of the contract. It shouldn't take me too long to become a sister, because I've got the experience, and I'd be quite happy having my own unit and running it the way I wanted – which means to decent standards. I wouldn't have nurses on my ward that didn't want to work for me. They'd be *out*. When I first started at Bart's one of the sisters said 'Don't bother to work on my unit unless you come here every day, and learn at *least* one thing new every day. You follow that rule for the rest of your nursing career, and you'll learn a lot in the end.' I do actually go out of my way to learn something new every day, and after seven years I *have* learnt quite a lot.

I don't think I'd go back into paediatrics, because to be a sister I'd have to become a registered sick children's nurse, which is *another* year's training, and I think after the conversion stint I'll have had it with courses.

And I'd like to get back to adults. Nursing children can be quite a strain. Some of those I'm dealing with at the moment haven't been given that long to live. Consequently they're extremely spoilt, and get away with murder. The parents will pander to their every single need, whereas I'd just like to get my hands on them and give them a good smack. The parents' attitude is understandable to a certain extent, but it still doesn't help when you've got a screaming child shouting 'Get out of my cubicle! Mummy! I want mummy! Go away! I'm not having anything to eat till mummy gets here.' Uh! Terrible! You get out quickly and shut the door.

What I'd really like is to have a male or female surgical ward to myself, either dealing with gastroenterology or cancer. You can do so much for your patients, and they respect you. You can help them get over their fear of surgery, and by good nursing care you can help them for the future, giving them psychological support and teaching them how to cope. The sort of surgery these people have to undergo often isn't very nice, and if you can give them the support and care they need they're so thankful. You can get a really good atmosphere going so that everybody's happy and contented.

But if I don't get my conversion course I shall leave. I don't know what I'll do, but I'll find *something*.

I feel I've got a lot to offer the profession if *only* I was given the chance, but that chance seems to be receding further and further into the distance, and I'm getting crosser and crosser. I'd be quite happy to walk into any intensive care unit in the country and just get on with it. I give of my best and keep myself up to date. It seems absolutely ludicrous to me that I have to go back and do another year of basic training – and I might not even get the chance to do that. Why can't we get an automatic conversion based on continuous assessment? If we've done well since we qualified, kept our knowledge up to date, and maybe done an extra course like I have, why can't we just take a short exam? Why should I spend my days off writing endless letters and getting answers saying 'No funds – Not interested – Write again next year' and all the rest of it? *All* the girls I know on *all* the courses at GOS have written dozens and dozens of letters and got nowhere. It's not good enough. They're going to lose a lot of nurses, and they'll be *good* nurses. A lot of enrolled nurses perform better than a lot of RGNs because we've got to *prove* we're worthwhile.

If I had my time again I'd work much harder for my O levels and my A levels. I'd have stuck it out and gone to college – to medical school. I'd very much like to have been a doctor. I'm sure I could have done it. But the careers advice we got at school was pretty appalling, and we weren't pushed enough, either.

People say to me 'Go back to school, and get your O levels and A levels, and go to medical school.' I could have done it, but it's too late now. I'm 24.

I'm a nurse, and that's what I'm going to be for the rest of my life, I suppose. I think I've got enough inside me to stick it out.

Chapter 4

TWO MIDWIVES

Molly Pritchard is a dauntingly-energetic community midwife aged 57. She is married to a headmaster and has five children. She went into nursing straight from school, but didn't train as a midwife until she was 45 and had finished producing babies of her own — an age at which most married nurses would feel they'd earned retirement from an onerous career. Her 'parish' covers a wide area of rural Cambridgeshire. When we'd finished talking she sent me home with a couple of jars of homemade jam. She's that kind of woman.

I think I always wanted to be a nurse. I did a pre-nursing course in the sixth form at my coed grammar school, and although I'd been offered a place in a London hospital they wouldn't take me before I was 18. I felt I just couldn't wait, so when I found the Luton and Dunstable Hospital would take girls who were a little bit younger I trotted off there, three months before my 18th birthday.

I joined the first ever group to go through their preliminary training school, because before September 1947 probationers had gone straight into the hospital. There's a photograph of us in a history of the hospital which has just come out. I'm the little fat one on the left.

I loved it. I was listening to three student nurses chatting together the other day, and I said 'You girls don't know you're born.' In my day we used to have to pull the beds out and sweep and dust and polish and then push them back again. As you got more senior, so you were elevated to the more superior tasks. The juniors swept and dusted. The next juniors polished the table. The next senior up had the privilege of polishing the sink and taps where the doctor washed his hands. That was *very* special. You had to have that absolutely gleaming.

We didn't have all the visiting we have now. Visiting days were Wednesdays and Sundays, and during visiting hours, depending on how senior you were, you did various chores – either cleaning the sluice, or tidying the linen cupboard, or doing the sterilisers and instruments and gallipots, or clearing out the medicine cupboard. Everything had to be arranged perfectly. I still try to keep my cupboards like that now, so that you can read the labels. If you did it wrong you had to go back and do it again.

When we were student nurses and went across to breakfast, the home sister would go into our rooms and pull the beds back to see if we'd made them properly. If we hadn't she'd strip them. You'd go back to your room in the coffee break. 'Oh, no!' You'd have to make it again. She'd make a note of whose beds she'd stripped, and go back during the day to see whether you'd made it again, and what time you'd done it. I still do my 'hospital corners' when I make beds at home.

We had *one* day off a week – no two-and-a-half *days* off – and very often on our one day we'd have lectures. We had to be in by ten, and if you wanted to go to the cinema, that was just tough luck. We *never* knew how the film ended, because we had to leave by half-past-nine to catch the bus.

The salary was an absolute pittance. The NHS hadn't come into being, and every month we used to go into the boardroom and file around to be given our pay packets, and just before Christmas we used to stop and take something out for the home sister's Christmas present, and something for the tutor's, and something for the assistant matron's, and something for the matron's. *Every* girl used to do that.

Then we'd line up to get a little present from the matron, which was usually a flannel, or a bar of soap, or something like that. She gave us all a present. She felt we were *her* girls. Her name was Miss

Redmond, and when I think of her I'm always reminded of Joyce
Grenfell singing 'Stately as a galleon, she sailed across the floor',
because she was a *very* large woman. She would have been a large
woman even if she'd only been four foot and five stone, but she
was about ten foot and 20 stone. She was a wonderful, wonderful
woman. She didn't stand for any nonsense. You knew *who* you
were, and *where* you worked, and *where* you belonged. You knew
exactly what you'd got to do.

It was very regimented, but I think it was good. You didn't have
little girls who've just started nursing calling ward sisters by their
Christian names and being overfamiliar with everybody.

I was getting something like £7 a month as a student nurse, but
board and lodging was all taken care of. We lived in and were fed
properly, and had just sufficient money to buy our black stockings
and our shoes, and a little bit left for toiletries and stamps and
Christmas presents. We were *very* poor, but that didn't matter,
because we were very wealthy in what we were doing. We had this
fantastic feeling of belonging. It was lovely.

There was none of this nonsense of cooking in kitchens,
and having your boyfriend living with you, and other people's
boyfriends using the bathroom in the nurses' home. Somebody
said to me recently 'We daren't even have a fire drill now. You
never know who you're going to flush out. You never know who's
living with who.'

When we qualified and got our belts, the sister tutor, Miss
Fletcher, glared at us and said 'There is no *safe* period, girls –
there is *no* safe period.' I don't know *why* she used to say that,
because men were definitely not part of our lives. You just didn't
have boyfriends. You didn't have *time* for boyfriends.

BACK TO SCHOOL

I always intended to be a midwife, but I met my husband before I
could do the training.

Then, 20 years later, I woke up one morning and thought
'Help! I'm going to be 45 any minute now, and if I don't do

it pretty soon nobody will want to train me. I'll be too old.'
I'd recently been doing some night duty on a maternity unit, and
because they couldn't recruit enough of their own full- time staff
all the midwives on at night were agency girls, and they weren't
native Britons. The mothers were all English, and they thought *I*
was the midwife, because I was the one who spoke the language.
I wasn't, of course, but I thought 'If those girls managed to train
successfully when they could hardly speak any English, then I'm
sure *I* can', so I looked around for somewhere willing to accept
a mature student.

By sheer coincidence I found that my old training school at
Luton would be quite interested. I think they thought it was a bit
of a giggle to have this old girl back again. I was in a group of about
12 girls, some of whom had just finished their general training,
but I wasn't aware of *any* age difference. They were absolutely
super to me. The only time I *was* made aware of my age was on
Mothering Sunday. We were doing our community training, and
I'd been out all night, and I came back in the morning absolutely
shattered, and they took me into the dining room, and there was
an enormous bouquet which they'd bought for me because they
were away from their *own* mothers.

I stayed at the hospital after finishing my training and did a
special care course, and I was the only one in my group offered
a staff job. I don't know whether that was because they thought I
was quite good, or if they thought 'Well, poor old soul, if we don't
offer her a post nobody else *will*. She's getting so ancient.'

I had this bee in my bonnet that I wanted to work in the
community. I felt that with my experience of a family spread
over the years I'd gleaned a useful bit of knowledge about life.
And I was so thankful that I did my midwifery training *after* I'd
had my babies.

But by this time I'd been going flat out for five years, and I
was rather exhausted. Just getting to work was a major exercise.
I'd been driving abroad, and had an overseas licence, but found I
had to take a test here, and I kept *failing*. So my husband used to
drive me into Hertford, and I'd get a bus from there to St Albans,
and then another bus to Luton, and then *another* bus up to the
hospital, and when I came home I had the whole rigmarole over

again. Looking back I don't know how I did it. I must have been terribly determined. Eventually I did pass my driving test, at the fifth attempt. I think it was a bad time in a woman's life to start doing something like that. I'd worn myself out, so I took a year off.

At the end of the year I thought 'What now?' I didn't want to go back as a part-time staff nurse, having *been* a sister, and I felt I really deserved a sister's post.

Intensive care was very much to the fore. I'd done the Luton course and got a hospital certificate, but that was only a local qualification. So I decided to do the special and intensive care course for the nationally-recognised certificate at the Sorrento Maternity Hospital in Birmingham, where they pioneered intensive care for premature babies. It was an extremely rewarding but very stressful six months, and I did begin to feel that that wasn't what I wanted to do.

Some nights we'd have *three* seriously-ill babies in incubators and on oxygen. You'd do the tipping and the suction and the physio and the intravenous feeding for one, and then move on and do the same for the next, and then for the next, and then back again to number one, and it went on like that all night, with ultraviolet light shining down on you, and you'd be peering through the glass of the incubators, with your spectacles on all the time to read the tiny print.

Night duty was horrendous, and I began getting headaches and feeling quite ill. They wanted people to stay on after the course, and I did consider it – keeping a room there, and travelling back and forth on the M1. I used to have the most hilarious adventures up and down the M1, slipping off the road, and getting bogged down in the snow, and being dug out by policemen. Oh dear!

But then the Cambridgeshire post came up and I applied and got it. At the interview I said 'Well, I promise you faithfully that I won't keep going off on maternity leave!'

WORKING THE PARISH

I'm employed by the Cambridgeshire Area Health Authority, and my patch contains 16 villages, but I work in conjunction with a group of general practitioners, and look after the pregnancies of all the ladies on their list. (I always refer to my clients as 'ladies' and not 'patients'. They're not ill.) I'm paired with a midwife working with another practice and we cover for one another on our days off. But I might have to cover for any of the other six midwives in our group, and about once a week I'm on call at night for the whole district.

The doctors I work with give me a lot of leeway and back me up to the hilt. They're happy to let me do what I think is needed and then let them know, whereas some of my colleagues have to ask their GP before they can send a baby into hospital for special care, or ask for a scan of a mother they think may have retained products, or whatever. So I *am* able to feel myself to be a practitioner in my own right – which a lot of midwives don't, and it makes them very unhappy. They feel very threatened.

I start my day at my desk at eight, and do paperwork and phoning until nine, and that's when my mothers can ring me, before I go out. Then I drive off to my patch.

Ideally you should do all your nursing first, but my ladies are so scattered that I mix the postnatals and the antenatals and the booking visits as I go round. Just going round my patch is 42 miles, and I can do anything up to 100 miles a day, back and forth, back and forth. I'm really like a vagabond, with everything floating around in the back of my car. In the winter you have to be prepared for every eventuality, so I have pieces of old cardboard, and shovels, socks, an extra coat, Wellington boots, and things like that, because sometimes you get totally stuck.

It gets particularly stressful on a Saturday or a Sunday, because then I'm out all day, and you don't have toilet facilities, and there's nowhere you can go, short of saying to a mother 'May I use your bathroom?' And that's something I can *never* bring myself to do. You literally grit your teeth. It *is* a painful experience.

We have to attend the newly-delivered mothers twice daily up to day three, then daily to day ten, and then at our discretion up to day 28. After that they're out of our hands, and the health visitor takes over. Sometimes, if I'm worried about a woman and think she may be suffering from postnatal depression or whatever, I make an excuse to go back and see her after I've finished with her

officially. I lend her a book or something, and then drop in later to
pick it up. The health visitor goes in twice after they've had their
babies, and then they go to a clinic, but they don't feel they have
anybody specifically to relate to. Today's mother hasn't got gran
or an Auntie Flo round the corner. It's awful if you've got some
kind of problem, and you keep seeing different people, and you
keep having to explain it all over again.

Last week I went to a girl who'd lost twins earlier this year and
had just had another miscarriage at 24 weeks. Yesterday I was
summoned to one of my mothers who'd just had an antepartum
haemorrhage and had lost a tremendous amount of blood. She'd
been whisked into the Rosie (the Cambridge maternity hospital)
and wanted to see *me* in the middle of a day – I thought I could
hardly manage what I'd got to do already, and *she* had to have
an hour of my time. Then I was told of another of my ladies
whose little girl had just died of cancer at the age of three. So in
the course of *one* week I had to deal with one mother who'd lost
a three-year-old, another who'd lost three babies in a year, and
another who'd had an early miscarriage. These women want to
talk their troubles out. It drains you emotionally, but *I* can't just
walk away from it, which is why I'm terribly slow at going round.
Some of my colleagues believe there's nothing you can't cope with
in the course of a ten-minute visit – you go in, and you go out.

We see the pregnant women once a month up to 28 weeks, and
then fortnightly up to 36 weeks, and then weekly. I do an antenatal
clinic at the surgery, and hold parentcraft and relaxation classes in
the villages, and whenever I can manage it I go into the Rosie to
deliver my mothers who've been taken in.

I do the antenatal clinics on my own, but a lot of my colleagues
do theirs with the doctor, which means they're just taking blood
pressures and testing urines, while the doctor does the palpating
and the rest. I say 'I'm not doing that. I'm a midwife. I like to get
my hands on my ladies.' So they'll see just me one week, and the
doctor the next.

I palpate them, I test their urine, I weigh them, I take their
blood pressure, I check their breasts, I check all the little bits
and pieces that need to be checked, and I make sure they
haven't got any varicose veins, or any other problems. If I'm

not happy with what I'm finding I'll ring the hospital and say 'I've got a lady here, and I'm pretty sure she's a breech. Can you have a look at her?'

The mothers appreciate this. They like to be in a room with a midwife. They can talk more frankly. They feel there are some intimate parts of their care they can discuss more freely with a woman, particularly if she's someone they've got to know right from the beginning of their pregnancy.

At the relaxation class I get them all to lie down on the floor and I put 'None but the weary heart' on the record player, and while that's playing I'm making the tea. I go round picking up an arm or a leg, and they don't bat an eyelid. I'm very pleased when this happens. Then I say 'Right, ladies – when you're ready – don't rush!' Meaning 'Hurry up!' And we have the talk and the tea, and they gradually get up, and some of them are yawning, and you *know* they've been to sleep. It's great!

When I'm on call, and if I get home late, I get the feeling that I never stop, because when I get in I have to make sure I have a clean dress and that my bag's at the ready so that I can leap out of bed and into my things and go off very quickly. I may be very, very tired and think 'Gosh, I must have a bath', but I can't wash my hair in case I'm called out, and I have to be quick in the bath, and I must do this, and I must do that.

I have to phone the hospital anytime after 11.30 pm, and they give me a list of all the day's discharges for our area. Then it's my job to phone the relevant midwives to make sure they visit these ladies the following day. I stay on call until eight in the morning, and have to deal with whatever turns up. We get paid the princely sum of £2 a night for being on call. I think it's £3 on a Saturday. I don't think you'd get a fish and chip meal for that. And when I think what the man charges just to make the *journey* to look at my washing machine! That's why the great British public doesn't really value us – because they know we're cheap, because we're *there* and we're cheap.

When I deliver one of my ladies in the hospital the delivery room becomes a little bit of the community. The hospital staff know that if I want them I'll shout, and it's good to have them around, but they don't interfere.

I'd be able to do more deliveries if I *worked* in a hospital as a staff sister, but my mothers would have to go through the hospital routine, and they'd be given this drug and that, and they'd be hooked up to monitoring equipment, and it would be all high-pressure stuff.

That's not how *I* want to deliver babies.

I want my ladies walking about – doing their ironing, finishing their knitting, scrubbing the floor if they want to, *jumping up and down* if they want to – and not getting up on to that delivery bed until it's time to get going with the active part.

Very few people have home confinements now. One of my colleagues in Cambridge does seem to get quite a few, but she's practically on top of the hospital, whereas I'm out in the villages. Mothers are indoctrinated. Some of them say to me 'Supposing something goes wrong?' They *expect* to bleed. They *expect* to have an epidural. They *expect* to have forceps. They *expect* to have a cut. Childbirth shouldn't *be* like that. I tell my ladies that childbirth is a normal, natural, physiological event, just like passing a motion. And then I tell them that if ever they pass a seven-pound motion they should come and talk to me about their diet.

If I was younger, and was going to have another baby, I'd *insist* on having it at home.

AWKWARD CUSTOMERS

I told somebody the other day that I don't look after my ladies – *they* look after me. We do have a great deal of fun. And we talk to each *other*. I don't talk *at* them. But it's not always like that.

I almost came to blows with one husband. He opened the door and said 'What time do you call this? I've just taken my wife's lunch up. She's been waiting all morning for you to come.' I said 'Well, I'm sorry Mr Whatever-his-name- was, it's impossible for me to give *everybody* the ten-o-clock visit.' And his wife was calling down the stairs saying 'Let Mrs Pritchard come up, then.'

I said 'Can I just pop up and see her?' He said 'It's extremely inconvenient.'

I said 'That's perfectly all right. You don't *have* to let me in. Perhaps we'll arrange for somebody else to come tomorrow. Perhaps I'd better go away.' He said 'I wish you *would*. My lunch is getting cold.'

There was a lady at Gamlingay who'd just had her second child and she needed to have her tummy checked. I told her I'd see her on Christmas Eve. 'Oh, don't come on Christmas Eve' she said. 'I've got masses of shopping to do. But I'll definitely be in on Christmas Day.'

'I'll be in the village' I said, 'but I only want to do essential calls. It's Christmas for me too, you know.'

'No' she said, 'please come on Christmas Day in the morning. That would suit me very much better. I'll definitely be here. But I won't be here on Christmas Eve.'

So I went on Christmas Day. I knocked on the door and heard this man say 'Who the hell's that?' He came down the corridor, and they'd got this glass front door. 'Christ!' he said. 'It's the bloody midwife!' He flung the door back and glared at me and I said 'And a Merry Christmas to you too!' I'd really had enough by then.

He said 'What the hell time do you call this? I didn't expect you to*day*.' I said 'Well, I'm sorry, but your wife specially asked me to come.'

So he shouted to his wife, and grudgingly let me in, and said 'We'll never get the bloody dinner at this rate.' He had a manfriend there, and off they went into another room, carrying their glasses. And there was this poor girl, who'd just had a baby, struggling in the kitchen.

I just glanced at the baby and said 'Right, my dear. Your own midwife will come and see you at the end of the week. I won't be back again.'

'I'm sorry', she sobbed. I said 'Don't worry about it. Forget it. My skin's thick.' I was furious.

Sometimes it's pouring with rain, and you have to find a place to park your car, and then walk to the house you're visiting, and you knock, knock, knock, and nobody answers. You then go back to the car, and write a note, and bring it to the house, and just as you're about to put it through the letterbox someone will open the door and say 'Oh, I *thought* it might be you!' And there you are, dripping wet, and you think 'Well, she *knew* I was coming.' If that happens ten times in a morning you can get a little disenchanted.

You do sometimes get rudeness. And then I think 'Well, was that *my* fault? Did I *invite* that?'

REFLECTIONS

Nowadays a woman who's just had a baby in hospital is asked 'Do you want to have a shower, love?' And she gets off the bed, but nobody *takes* her. She staggers to the loo. She staggers to the shower. If she doesn't feel like it, and *if* there's an auxiliary around, she'll get a blanket bath. The midwife is too busy.

I see midwifery as doing the whole thing. When you deliver a woman you look after her. You bath her. You put her comfortable. You make her a tray of tea and take it in to her. You look after the husband as well. Then you bath the baby. That's part of the job.

Not any more. Everybody's rushing. If you're trained in midwifery you deliver babies. Somebody else – an SEN or an auxiliary – will go and bath the mother.

I don't think self-discipline does anybody any harm. I can't help comparing the stamina and staying power of people of my age group with that of these 21-year-olds. When we're doing something we just keep going till we've finished. They *must* go off. They're very much into making sure they get their breaks. They watch the clock. And when it's time to go off, they're *off*. There's no staying over to finish a task. That's it! They've done their time. They're *going* I think it's a shame. Nursing is a commitment.

As soon as most women get pregnant they hand their bodies over, and they're so *bovine* about it. They let people lead them along by their noses. They do what they're told. They take the view that they don't know anything about it, so therefore *we* must know better, and if the consultant says this, that, or the other shall be done, they quite happily submit to it.

And then you get the 'fringe' women, the ones I used to call the 'lentil eaters.' You get a lot of those in Cambridge. They're into natural feeding. They have *respect* for their bodies, and they're not *going* to be conveyor-belted. They're not *going* to put up with needles and drips and pessaries and episiotomies and forceps. They're going to do their own thing. They've got a far healthier and far more natural attitude toward childbirth.

I tell my mothers that if they decided to go in for a marathon they'd practise for it. They can't expect to get pregnant and just carry on with everything they've been doing. A lot of these girls don't even stop work at 28 weeks, specially now the maternity allowance has been changed. They're becoming the new poor, and they carry on working as long as they possibly can.

I'm not surprised to find that when they stop work at 33 weeks they have their babies at 34 or 35. They haven't given themselves a chance. They have tiny babies, and bad labours, and come home feeling absolutely worn out.

If you want to do something properly, you've got to prepare for it.

Some of these girls conceive their babies very easily. They beget very easily. But once they've begotten, they don't know what to do with them. They dress them up in their little frilly frocks, and they walk them around, and take pictures of them, and give them to the children to play with. It's absolutely astonishing.

We tend just to look after the pregnant uterus.

You can spend hours discussing breastfeeding, but it comes right down to one basic thing. If a mother wants to do it, she will, and if she doesn't you can talk till you're blue in the face, and she won't.

Even when I did my midwifery at Luton 15 years ago midwives were delivering breeches. We were taught the various manoeuvres, and we jolly well used to have to know how to do it. You could have an undiagnosed breech, and there'd be nobody else around, and you just had to get on with it.

It's 'Hands off breeches' now. If there's a breech, or if there are twins, you *know* the midwife won't get that delivery. The doctor has to do it. We're not the professionals we were.

In the five years I've been working in Cambridgeshire I've seen lots and lots of changes.

We've got non-nurses and non-midwives *managing* nurses and midwives, and they haven't a clue how we work. They don't understand the stresses we're under. They don't understand doctors' pressures. They're there to save money, that's their prime object. It's all very well for somebody with managerial experience to arrange things on paper, but you can't *arrange* people on paper.

The little hospital in Royston is under threat of closure. We've just had the maternity unit closed down there. It only had six beds, but it played a very, very valuable part in the community.

I'm very old-fashioned in my approach to my patients and my colleagues and my work, and I feel that the one-to-one relationship is what we need. And we're not getting it.

A FINAL AMBITION

I saw in my *Nursing Chronicle* the other day that they're wanting midwives to work for VSO in West Africa. I said to my husband 'I know what I'm doing next year. When Alan goes off to university, I'm going out to West Africa to look after pregnant women for a couple of years, because they *take* old people, you know.'

I'd like to do that.

Jilly Rosser is not a nurse. She is an independent midwife with a small private practice in north London. She qualified in 1979 after a two-year course (now three) in pure midwifery at Derby City Hospital, which was, at the time, the only centre in the country offering such training. She is fiercely proud of her unalloyed state.

Ms Rosser received nationwide publicity in September 1987 after being suspended from practice by the North-East Thames Regional Health Authority. This followed allegations of 'professional misconduct' arising from an incident which most people would look upon as having demonstrated her common sense, initiative and excellent clinical judgment, rather than any kind of imperfection.

At the time of writing no fewer than six independent midwives are 'under investigation', which fact, in view of their thinness on the ground, suggests that the very existence of freelancers might be a source of irritation to the midwifery establishment, so that their performance tends to be observed in an unusually sharp and carping fashion.

I'm a direct-entry midwife, with no nursing qualification, and I did the pure midwifery course specifically because I didn't *want* to be a nurse. I wanted a job in which I was an independent practitioner, which I don't see nursing as being. I'm interested in caring for childbearing women, and in working with *women* as opposed to *men* and women. A lot of the older midwives were trained like that. Then the opportunity all but dried up, but it's about to start all over again, and there'll be several places doing it in a couple of years. They're just getting the curriculum organised.

The training was disappointing. We had almost no clinical teaching, and I did most of my learning from textbooks. We weren't supernumerary on the wards, so we spent a lot of our time making beds, catheterising people, escorting women in the antenatal clinic – all the normal duties. I did get *experience*, because we just went and *did* things, and learnt by watching other people, and by asking questions, and by making mistakes, and hoping they weren't bad ones. We were treated very badly, just as an extra pair of hands, and somebody without opinions.

You end up as a state certified midwife, but after I'd qualified I soon realised I didn't want to work in the NHS. As I've said, I went into midwifery because I wanted to be an independent practitioner, but if you work in a hospital you're completely bound by hospital policies. Each woman is considered as almost the property of a particular consultant and you carry out that consultant's policies, instead of treating her as the individual you see before you and giving her the care you think appropriate to *her*. I had no interest at all in working like that.

At the end of the '70s we were at the height of the tendency toward routine and irresponsible intervention, and the use of unevaluated procedures. This was causing an awful lot of hardship and *suffering* to women, and I didn't want to be any part of it.

So I left the country and did something completely different.

ROUND THE WORLD

I went to Yemen and worked for a small voluntary organisation, the Catholic Institute for International Relations, as a trainer of traditional birth attendants.

I lived in a small and very remote village in the mountains and started a project which also included the training of primary health-care workers. They had a very high incidence of perinatal mortality, and we were attempting to train the women who were already *attending* women in labour to make their work safer and better. We were teaching them to give fairly rudimentary antenatal care, which they hadn't been doing.

Anaemia was quite a severe problem, so we got them to give out iron tablets. We trained them to refer any serious problems of pregnancy, but there weren't many of those. We taught them to feel the position of the baby, so that if it was in a bad position, like a transverse lie, we'd know about it *before* labour was well advanced. We trained them to cut and tie the cord in a sterile way. We gave them a few basic guidelines on the handling of retained placentas or bleeding. They were given ergometrine tablets to use. But one of the main things we taught them was the advantage of breastfeeding, and the danger of bottle-feeding, because badly managed bottle-feeding is the biggest cause of infant mortality in Yemen.

I was there to teach, and not to do clinical work, but I did get called to emergencies, and I didn't have *any* backup. I was the end of the line, which is not a pleasant situation to be in. I had some equipment, and if I got called to a retained placenta or a haemorrhage I'd have the drugs and the drips. I never lost a woman to that. But I hadn't been trained to use forceps, and

I obviously couldn't do caesarian sections, so if a woman was in delayed labour, and if that was what she really required, she died. You couldn't get her to an obstetrician. The nearest road was five hours away. And anyway, the women wouldn't travel, and they wouldn't have men examine them. It was a very traditional part of the country. So the women would die of delay in labour, and sometimes from bleeding.

A lot of children died from diarrhoea. Sometimes infectious diseases like measles and whooping cough would wipe out whole villages. They had various traditional treatments which worked some of the time, but they had a fatalistic outlook, and very much left things up to God.

I left Yemen after two-and-a-half years. I wrote a report for UNICEF on the traditional birth-attendant training programme in Sudan, and then went round the world, staying with midwives across North America and Australasia, studying different working methods and situations, and learning a great deal. That took the best part of a year.

Then I came back here and spent another year on a diploma course in primary health-care education, because while in Yemen I'd felt my lack of teaching ability.

After that I got a job in Guinea-Bissau training the *trainers* of traditional midwives – training the *trained* midwives in how and what to teach. The health problems were completely different from those in Yemen. There was an awful lot of neonatal tetanus, which you never saw in Yemen, but they all breastfed their babies, so I didn't even have to *mention* bottles.

That lasted 18 months, because I met my husband and became pregnant and came back here to have my baby.

PRIVATE PRACTICE

I've been working as an independent midwife since September 1986. I didn't plan to set up in practice, but a pregnant friend of a friend was looking for a midwife just when a group of independent practitioners had left the area, and I was asked if I'd take her on, and thought 'Well, why not?' Word got around among people involved in the birth movement that an independent midwife was working in north London again, and I began to get referrals from birth classes.

Now there are four of us. It's really going up again. It's great. Two work together as partners, and I and the other one cooperate; we're not partners, but we cover for one another.

You don't have to be approved or get permission in order to start a private practice. So long as you're a registered certified midwife you just have to write to the supervisor of midwives for the relevant health authority saying 'I'm practising in your area.' She then becomes your supervisor for any cases you take on. So the midwifery structure works for all independent midwives, even though we're operating outside the NHS. I'm actually registered with several authorities – Haringey, Bloomsbury, Islington, Hampstead – all around.

When you take on your first case in a district they ask to check your equipment. After that you notify them every time you book a woman, giving her address, saying who her GP is, and noting a few other details, and then you just get on with it.

Quite a lot of women come to me after they've tried the NHS and have been disappointed. In fact, the first thing I do is check that they *have* considered all the alternative forms of care, because I'm not trying to poach from the NHS.

So when a woman comes to me I find out what she wants. Whether she'd like to be booked into a hospital for the delivery. Whether she wants me to deliver her at home. Whether she gets on well with her GP and would like him to share the antenatal care, or whether she doesn't and would rather I did everything. Whatever she wants, that's what she gets. But I've yet to have a woman who wanted her GP at the birth. They all specifically say they don't want *any* doctors at the birth. And if she *doesn't* want the GP present, there's no more to be said.

I've had two women booked with me who were going to have their babies in hospital anyway, but they wanted continuity of care, and that's the main reason for women employing independent midwives. Even when they've got *lovely* community midwives – and there are plenty of lovely community midwives – they don't know who's going to be delivering their babies. But I make a contract with my clients and say that, short of breaking a leg or having to attend another labour, I'll be there at the birth.

There are some health authorities – Westminster is a good example – who will give independent midwives an honorary contract so that they can work as midwives within the hospital and conduct deliveries. And that's very nice for a woman with a potential problem; there's expert help immediately available should it be needed, but if all goes well her own midwife can see her through. Other hospitals won't do that, and then you're simply there as a knowledgeable support and advocate, and you just stand around and *talk*. But *that's* important.

Most of us don't like to book more than four women a month. You have to be on call from about 36 weeks, but plenty of women go two weeks overdue, and by that time you're waiting for the next one to go into labour. So you're *perpetually* on call, 24 hours a day and seven days a week, which is exhausting.

It's the postnatals who are so time consuming, especially if you're visiting twice a day, and you have two or three living in opposite directions, and there's a lot of traffic. That's why we keep our lists small.

SUSPENSION

I was delivering a woman who I'd had booked with me from about 16 weeks. I'd shared the antenatal care with her GP.

She went into labour and had a normal baby. The placenta delivered normally and everything seemed fine. Then her condition began to deteriorate.

I called the hospital to say we might be coming in, but she recovered, so I called again to say we *weren't* coming. Then she deteriorated again and I said 'I really think you ought to go into hospital', but she said 'I don't want to. Will you call the GP?' So I said 'OK.'

I tried calling the GP, but it was Sunday afternoon and it was some 20 minutes before I learnt he wasn't answering his bleep. She was getting worse, and before the 20 minutes was up I'd already decided she *would* have to go in. We took her to the Whittington in her own car with her partner driving. It's only about five minutes drive away, and with no traffic on a Sunday afternoon we got there very quickly.

As we got her out of the car she passed an *enormous* clot. They had a drip in her arm within moments. She was *very* well cared for. They stopped the bleeding and diagnosed a cervical tear. They took her to the theatre, stitched her up, gave her blood, and she recovered.

I went home thinking 'Well, it was unfortunate, but a cervical tear isn't something anybody can *predict*, and you can't know it's *happening*.' It's extremely rare, and in her case I couldn't tell that it *had* happened, because she wasn't bleeding per vagina. She was forming a clot at the *top* of the vagina, and the uterus was contracted. It was a *very* unusual case, and I'm sure I'll never see one like it again.

So I hadn't felt I'd been in *any* way responsible for such an unfortunate thing happening, and I thought I'd acted properly and done the right thing. It didn't occur to me that anyone else would think otherwise. I went home, and did another delivery, and then this whole disciplinary procedure started.

They started saying that I should have called the obstetric flying squad, which is, of course, the ideal way for a woman to be transported – no doubt about it – but I was extremely worried by the fact that she was *deteriorating*. The flying squad has to organise personnel and equipment before it sets out, so there's quite a lot of preparation time, even if everything goes smoothly.

I have a Hampstead couple booked with me, and they had their first baby at home with an independent midwife in 1986. The mother had a serious postpartum haemorrhage with a retained placenta, and the midwife called the flying squad, and it took an hour-and-a-quarter to get there. So they arrived at the Royal Free, which was only half-a-mile down the road, one-and-a-half hours after the call for help was made. The woman had lost four pints of blood, and was nearly unconscious.

Now she's pregnant again, and I've *told* her she's at some risk of having the same thing happen, but she's determined to go ahead at home, and to be transferred to hospital if necessary. But in view of her last experience she *insists* that if it comes to that she should be taken in by private car.

That story was one of the things that helped me make up my mind. Quite apart from the possibility of a long delay, there isn't a flying squad at the Whittington, which was only five minutes away. They come from University College Hospital, or from various places which are 20 minutes away.

So I got her to medical aid the quickest way I knew how, and I'd do the same thing again tomorrow, even if I knew I'd get into trouble for it. In fact there's no rule which says the midwife must call the flying squad.

I was suspended on the spot by the regional health authority, on the grounds that I'd broken the rule which obliges us to call medical aid if there's an emergency or any deviations from the normal, which is, of course, quite right. But what's the difference between *calling* medical aid and *going* to medical aid? There is *none*. It should be a matter for the midwife's judgment. *I* was there. *I* saw the woman's condition. And *I* thought the most appropriate thing to do was to take her in by private car.

So I've been suspended from practice and lost my livelihood on the say-so of *another* midwife – the regional nursing officer – who happens to think differently. I've never talked to her, she's never asked to speak to me, and I've not been able to explain myself.

My case was considered just the other day by the English National Board of Nurses, Midwives and Health Visitors. They could have decided there was no case to answer, and have reinstated me, but they've decided there *is* a case to answer, and I've now got to wait for a full hearing before the Professional Conduct Committee of the UKCC, which won't take place until May 1988. Meanwhile I stay suspended.

The English Board only considers written evidence. I put in my side of the story, but of all the people who've been deciding my case so far, not *one* single one has spoken to me. It's Draconian, and quite unnecessary. There has to be *some*thing to protect women and babies. There *are* midwives who go to work drunk, or who misuse drugs, or who seem to be completely incompetent, and there must be a mechanism for suspending dangerous midwives. But the present system's wrong.

I'm not the only person this has happened to. Quite a lot of midwives have been suspended wrongly, by use of the wrong procedure, or for the most ridiculous reasons.

I haven't been struck off the register – yet. I've just been suspended by the regional authority, and if I wanted to move house and go and live in another region – which I *don't*, thank you very much – I could go on practising, at least until May. Fortunately I have a part-time job working 20 hours a week for a charity called the Midwives Information and Resource Service. I edit their information pack, which helps to keep midwives up to date, so I do have a little money coming in. I've had considerable publicity and an awful lot of support. I think there'll be changes.

(In fact, Ms Rosser's case dragged on through the summer with a final hearing expected in September 1988.)

STATE OF THE ART

Midwifery is in a pretty bad state at the moment, but I think it's reached rock bottom and will soon be on the way up.

Midwives aren't able to practise as practitioners. If you're in a hospital you're bound by the consultant's policy, and that's a very unsatisfactory way of working. Midwives are trained to take responsibility for normal childbirth, but they're not, in fact, permitted to do this.

Working conditions are very, very difficult. Apart from Draconian management, which appears here and there, there's an enormous shortage of midwives, which adds to the stress on those who remain. The official line is that a woman in labour should have the sole attention of a midwife. Very few places manage that now, though. There's usually one for every two or three women in labour, which is utterly unacceptable. A lot of midwives want to give continuity of care, and that's what women want. Women should be able to know that one or other of a small group of midwives will see her during the antenatal period, be with her during labour, and look after her postnatally. She should have the opportunity to get to know all of them, and they her. It's not much to ask that someone you *know* delivers your baby, but the health service in this country can't provide that, and I think it's shameful.

It's wrong that most midwives are nurses. Nurses are trained to carry out doctors' orders and care for the sick. Most of the time midwives aren't carrying out doctors' orders, and we're not caring for the sick, so nursing is a very inappropriate model for midwifery. That *is* changing, because more and more places will be offering pure midwifery training within the next few years, and that's a great change for the better.

At the moment the only way you can be promoted as a midwife is to move out of the clinical field and go into management. It's crazy. All our most experienced midwives are being lost to the business of childbearing, and lost to the teaching of students. Anyway, what's another midwife doing telling me what to do? The hierarchical structure isn't appropriate to midwifery at all, and it's one of the things that stops the Pay Review Body giving midwives a completely different deal to nurses. I think we *will* get a new grading structure which will allow us promotion while staying on our real job.

The pay's inadequate. It's an extremely responsible job. We have, after all, the life of the mother and child in our hands. Yet we're paid about the same as a London copy typist, and plenty of secretaries get paid much more. A staff midwife gets £7,500. I think the starting pay should be about £12,000.

All the independent midwives I know would much rather be working within the NHS, but we simply can't operate there in the way we'd wish.

Chapter 5

TROUBLED MINDS

Our institutions for the long-term care of the dependent old and the mentally disabled have a shameful reputation. For over 20 years now a succession of official reports have told of abysmal physical conditions, filthy toilets, poor food, a lack of any kind of stimulating occupation, gross overuse of tranquillising drugs, callous handling, and often, even, overt cruelty. It does not have to be like that.

Steve Goodwin is a registered mental nurse and currently a social services divisional manager in Blackburn, responsible for the district's public and private homes for the old and the disabled. He is a maverick, but a maverick possessed of so much energy and conviction that increasing numbers of his nursing colleagues are being seduced into sharing his admirable and unorthodox views. As a result of their experience in psychiatric hospitals he and a partner founded a movement which they call Cosmic Nursing – a kind of invisible college devoted to spreading the novel idea that the failing old and the mentally impaired harbour the same sense of selfhood, and experience the same appetites, emotions and even ambitions, as the rest of us, and that if these dispositions are catered for, the quality of their lives can be vastly improved.

He feels a profound respect (unusual among the young) for
the past achievements and struggles of men and women now
retired from the fray, and his office in Blackburn is hung with
reproductions of World War I recruiting posters – a seeming
tribute to those Old Contemptibles who are still alive.

I can't really remember what made me interested in nursing. I'd
left school at 16 with a few O levels, and tried my hand at various
jobs. I thought perhaps I'd like to be a fireman, but although I'd be
a dab hand at fires in bungalows, firemen have to climb ladders,
and I'm absolutely terrified of heights. Anyway, I started training
as a psychiatric nurse at 18 and knew right away and without
doubt that that was what I wanted to do.

Even though I'd no preconceived ideas, I realised from the start
– from my first ward experience – that my attitude clashed with
that of the people in authority. I was on a ward for the elderly
mentally ill, and the objective was just to keep people tolerably
clean and avoid problems. It was a game ending in a goalless draw.
You were reassured that everybody was happy in their own little
world, whereas I felt that the little world they were in was a far
from happy environment. Full stop!

There was a mixture of people on that ward. People who'd had
a mental illness all their *life* and grown old inside the institution,
and others who'd developed a dementia but who had once led
very *interesting* lives. Many were Great War veterans, or had held
key positions as architects or doctors or whatever. And they'd all
been thrown into this human scrapyard together, where they were
treated almost as if they were aliens; as if they hadn't *had* any past
history, or that if they had it was irrelevant, because *now* they were
just the way they were.

The standard of care expected of you as a nurse was much lower
than if you'd been dealing with any other member of the public. But
I felt, even at that very early stage, that I wanted them to be treated
like the rest of us – that they should be dressed properly and have
their own clothes, that they should enjoy good meals, properly
served. And people looked at me as much as to say 'Oh, it will soon
wear off. By the time he's done his three years' training, he'll have

forgotten these Utopian ideals.' I didn't see them as Utopian. It takes no more effort, in many ways, and certainly doesn't *cost* any more, to provide good care rather than bad care. It's a matter of attitudes.

I felt that the 30 or 40 students who'd come on the same block as me had been put on elderly-care wards to *start* their training on the grounds that it really didn't matter how they performed since they were only handling old people. And most of them were eager to get into acute psychiatry, with flashing lights and psychotherapy and so on – to be members of the psychiatric SAS, as it were. I, on the other hand, felt this to be an area needing the greatest amount of skilled care.

That wasn't the general view. The charge nurses and ward sisters on elderly-care wards were seen as a lower class of the profession, and most students were quite sure that was the one job they *didn't* want to end up doing. Although I very much enjoyed working in acute psychiatry, I took an opposite view.

I made friends with some of the people I nursed, which was very much frowned upon. I'm just talking about casual friendships, and I didn't allow it to happen with the women, for obvious reasons, but I felt that so long as you kept the relationship under control there was nothing wrong in treating your patients as if they were fellow human beings. In the end that paid handsome dividends, and it was basically the way I learned my psychiatry, because I was a terrible person for studying. I felt I got a lot more out of sitting down and talking to people. It's only after you've formed a deeper relationship with people that they're willing to tell you how they actually *feel* about their illness.

I never opened a textbook in the whole of my three years' training. The only text I've ever used is Giles' book of hospital cartoons, which is a classic commentary on the relationship between nurses and patients. When it came to the exams I was able to give *practical* answers to situations, based on people's real-life experiences, and I got a gold medal in my RMN finals.

ON THE JOB

I applied for a job staffing on a long-stay ward for the elderly mentally ill (EMI), which is where angels fear to tread. It was regarded as a career graveyard. As a matter of fact most of my contemporaries ended up in EMI as well, despite having opted for acute psychiatry or rehabilitation or industrial therapy, or whatever, because that's where most of the vacancies were.

I used to enjoy taking a lot of the patients out to all sorts of places. That wasn't actually frowned on, but nobody could see the *point* of it, because they were regarded as second-class citizens – *worse* than second-class citizens – who lived in a bizarre, alien world of their own, so that they didn't fit into normality. Faced with normality they might disintegrate.

There were the usual 'lunatics' outings' to the country, or a café, or a concert, and all the other institutional nonsense, and the local pub had a special room for people from the hospital. But I was more interested in taking people into *ordinary* situations, like ordinary pubs, where they'd be treated as ordinary people, as if they were elderly friends or relatives of mine. I'd take one or two home with me. My colleagues couldn't see the point.

Later I went to a very backward large psychiatric hospital in Devizes, and again chose to work on a typical long-stay 'back ward' for the EMI, which was just a continuation of everything I'd already seen. Everybody there had basically been written off. The décor was abysmal, nobody had their own clothes, and they very rarely got out. The staff were all good, kind, well-meaning people, and they worked hard and cared a lot, but the end result of all their effort was often just desolation and despair. It seemed sad to me that people should work so hard for so long and achieve the opposite to what they'd set out to achieve, and not *realise* it.

We talk about psychiatric patients having a lack of insight into their illnesses. I felt that *nurses*, including myself, had a lack of insight into the way we acted and worked and what we *did* with the day.

I was then 22, and I moved back to Blackburn as the only charge nurse on a small long-stay EMI ward which was part of a psychiatric unit attached to a large general hospital. This was my opportunity to sit down and plan my own philosophy of care, because in my previous posts I'd been a staff nurse and a deputy, and although I'd been pretty much left to get on with things and work according to my own ideas, much of what I did would be undone by people on other shifts. At Blackburn I was lucky to have a nurse manager who also had ideas and a wish to see the place prosper.

The ward held a mixture of people who just didn't go together. There were a lot of elderly people with dementia, including Great War veterans who'd fought with the East Lancs Regiment – people who'd led *real* lives and had great histories behind them. Tremendous. Very colourful characters. Then there were young men with Huntingdon's chorea who had some insight into the fact that they were facing a terrible death. And we had men in their 30s with alcoholic dementia, and one or two who'd been brain-damaged in road accidents.

The whole aim was just to look after these people until they died, and keep them out of trouble in the meantime. Don't let them stray into other wards. So long as we made sure they didn't get in anybody else's way it didn't really matter *what* happened. If people died of a chest infection, or some other physical illness, that was *fine*. But don't let them fall through a window, or get run over by a bus. Don't let anything untoward happen. There was no aim toward anything *positive*.

There was a lack of facilities. There was a lack of *everything*. There was certainly no *medical* input. Nobody was going to get better. There was no talk of anybody *ever* getting better. The doctors would regularly make their rounds and prescribe tranquillisers, either because they'd found somebody creating a bit of a disturbance, or just because that's what the nurses expected of them. That's what the nurses reckoned the doctors were *there* for.

By this time I'd already come to feel that medication is rarely the right policy. I'd worked on a secure unit where I'd seen large quantities of tranquillisers administered, as pills or by injection, and on the whole they simply didn't *help*. They provide a temporary solution to the problem posed by an awkward patient, but a much broader and deeper approach is needed, and their physical effects are very detrimental. Elderly people lose all their characteristics. They become completely colourless. They become aliens. They dribble and can't speak properly, and stagger, and are even more confused. I felt it was totally inhuman to *do* that to people, specially at the whim of individuals who just happen to have a badge on their lapels.

This was an open unit, and my ward was very noisy with a lot of activity going on, and the main problem was that people kept wandering off. They were continuously walking out of the unit and through the hospital grounds, and much further. The task of trying to keep them in was never-ending, from the moment they got up till nightfall. It was like keeping goal. The only way we could have done it was to lock the door, or sedate them heavily, or restrain them physically. So because we felt we couldn't *stop* them going out, we asked ourselves whether we were even right to *try*.

I'd appointed three or four auxiliaries who'd not done any nursing before, including a postman who'd never been in a hospital in his life. I wanted to get some people on the ward who hadn't any preconceived ideas about helping people. We sat down and looked at what we were doing, and why, and really tested our own attitudes.

The first thing we decided was that a lot of received wisdom about the elderly, and nursing, and psychiatry, and care generally, is inaccurate and basically untrue. And one wrong belief was that if you let elderly people wander they'd be run over by a steam roller, or turn out to be mass rapists, and anarchy would break out on the streets. But when you looked at the facts you found that these people who had wandered out – usually in pyjamas, or in shirt-sleeves in the middle of winter – *hadn't* come to any harm, even though by all means they should have done.

So we decided that we'd actually encourage *some* people to wander – those who had road sense – even though they might be quite confused. We'd see where they went and what they did, and then base our care on the facts we found out, instead of on pre-conceived opinions. We'd already diminished their tranquillisers, sometimes down to nothing, so they were now more rational, and we'd taken them walking with a nurse to various places every day, so they were quite physically fit. They were very humorous and colourful characters. Then we bought them the proper equipment to go out wandering – proper shoes, ski jackets, flat caps – and we gave them food for their pockets.

We did it properly. We discussed it with relatives, and with the police, and with the taxi firm that held the contract to the hospital. We took their photographs and made a note of what they were wearing when they got up in the morning. We didn't say 'Come on! Off you go!' If they were settled, and didn't want to go out, then they didn't. But if someone had wandered we'd keep a record of where he was found or where we'd picked him up. So, after a while, if someone hadn't returned by a certain time, and we hadn't been told by someone where he was, we'd be able to say to the police 'This is what he's wearing, and he's likely to be in that district.' And we all had cars, and would go out ourselves looking for people who hadn't come back.

Usually they went home, or to their relatives, or to where they used to live. Most of them would end up at the house they'd *last* lived in. Sometimes it had been sold, but we'd talk to the people there and say 'This person might end up on your doorstep', or the neighbours would ring up and say 'He's arrived here.' There was one man who they'd give a pair of hedge-cutters to, and he used to cut all the hedges in the *street*, so *everybody* was happy.

People generally ended up in the same place. There were one or two occasions when they didn't, and went *completely* astray. But nobody ever came to any harm.

Although at the time this scheme didn't seem immensely important, it actually set a precedent in nursing, because it demonstrated that the excuse for keeping these people shut in, which everybody had been using for donkeys' years – that if you let them out they'd come to great harm – was actually a myth.

A lot of these people did have quite severe dementia, but on the whole everybody improved dramatically. We got people moving who hadn't walked anywhere for years. Nobody had *shown* that they couldn't walk. It was just *assumed* that they couldn't do this, that, or the other thing. So we started to look at everybody individually, and found that if they had glasses, if they had teeth, if they had hearing aids, if they had *practice* in walking, if they had confidence and were given the chance to have a go, then they altered and could do all sorts of things.

That change in attitude snowballed. Care staff had always been used to the negative aspects of the job, without seeing some of the very positive opportunities.

Now, just down the corridor from us was a ward run in the old style, where the philosophy was 'These people are old and sick and disabled. They couldn't cope with a coach trip. And anyway, we're far too busy.' But their busy-ness consisted of treating pressure sores, making beds and caring for physical disorders. People were clinically depressed on that ward. They were *frightened*. And it was a vicious circle, because the more trapped the patients were the more disorders they developed. It was a Catch 22 situation. There's no reason why somebody with a pressure sore shouldn't sit in a coach for 20 minutes, or lie on the back seat if necessary, rather than be sitting on a vinyl chair in a geriatric ward.

We didn't take the *very* frail out, but the decrease in physical disorders was phenomenal. Forget about your disorder. Sometimes the best thing for somebody with a chest infection is to get out and enjoy a breath of fresh air. People kept cooped up often develop illnesses anyway, because hospital wards are commonly rife with infection.

We encouraged relatives to feel that they were part and parcel of the care team, and they could become more important than the nurses and other professionals. We'd actually collect relatives to visit, because often they were elderly ladies who were pretty frail themselves. We used to tell them that while their men would never again be able to go back home to live, that didn't mean they couldn't have them for the odd weekend, or for a day, or for an *hour*. A lot of relatives took us up on that. They would bake for the afternoon, and we'd deliver the patient, and we had such good rapport that sometimes if someone wasn't well enough to go home, and the baking had been done, we'd say 'We can't bring your husband today. He's got diarrhoea. Is it OK if somebody else comes?' And they'd say 'By all means.'

When someone died on the ward we'd always attend the funeral, and sometimes *arrange* the funeral, and we continued to care for the elderly relatives. We didn't feel that death should be the signal to sound the retreat. They were prospective clients, anyway.

We tried very hard to enjoy the job, which was totally unheard of in nursing. You're not *meant* to enjoy nursing. You're meant to walk around with that beetle-browed look, appearing to be extremely busy. You always have to be *doing* things. Whether they're constructive things is irrelevant, so long as you *look* busy.

COSMIC NURSING

After working in Blackburn for a while I got myself seconded to the Wirral for six months to do an English National Board course on the care of the elderly, and it was from there that I wrote up the philosophy of Cosmic Nursing.

The course was incredible. It was supposed to be a specialist course on how to look after old people, but I don't think I actually learnt *anything*. We were wandering through elderly care wards and social services homes and going out with health visitors, but nobody said anything constructive. There was nothing about the *attitude* we ought to have toward the job, which I'd always felt was the biggest problem in nursing. The biggest limitation elderly and disabled people suffer is in the minds of *other* people.

While I was there I met a lad called Paul Mangan. He was an enrolled general nurse, but he'd worked in psychiatry on elderly-care wards, and we found our ideas were so similar that we decided to join forces.

They wouldn't let us work together on the course because I think we wreaked havoc wherever we went, for the simple reason that we'd agreed that we wouldn't stand by bad practice. We were seeing things which were enough to make anybody weep. If somebody said 'This is the way you do *this*' and we thought they were wrong, we'd say 'No, it *isn't*.' You don't make yourself popular by criticising other people's nursing. It's like criticising other people's driving. But it has to be done, because the cost of bad nursing is enormous – not in money, but in the quality of patients' lives.

We got ourselves into a bit of trouble, I more than Paul, because he was an enrolled nurse and inclined to do what he was told, whereas I was a charge nurse, and when you're in charge of a ward you're there to represent a group of people who very often can't represent themselves. Sometimes, for example, a junior hospital doctor would come on to the ward ten minutes before a ward round and ask about the patients so that he could scribble something on the notes before the consultant appeared. Because nurses like to be liked they'd usually cooperate with this kind of cover-up, but I wouldn't. I'd say 'You ought to have your own opinions about these people. If you don't even know their *names*, that's your problem.' Then the consultant would say 'You haven't written anything in the notes. Why not?' And they'd panic, and eventually you got them to realise that you expected these old people to be treated with the same sort of care as any other patients. When you do that kind of thing in a hospital where you're not known it can cause problems. And it *did* cause problems. We became unpopular.

But at the end of the six-month course I presented Cosmic Nursing as my project, and it was very well received. I called it Cosmic Nursing because I wanted to sell the idea that the care of these old people is an exciting and interesting and all-embracing task, and not the boring, insignificant chore it's generally supposed to be.

I wrote up my ideas as a collection of jottings, some of them in verse even. It wasn't a formal thesis. Word of it got around, and people began to ask for copies, so that in the end about 1500 went out. Eventually the *Nursing Times* picked it up, and they got me and Paul to do a series, and in that same year we won a National Nursing Award, which is a prize given by the *Nursing Times* and 3M for contributions to nursing practice.

Cosmic Nursing tries to look at every aspect of care for the elderly. We try to point out how complex and skilled the job is if it's to be done well. Anybody can do it badly.

It's *feelings* that are important. Most nurses have a psychiatric disorder when it comes to appreciating the feelings of people. Some staff will get elderly people up in the morning without giving them their teeth. If I said to my staff 'Let's have your teeth, and you can have them back at the end of the day' do you think they'd part with their dentures? They'd go hysterical.

I once locked a woman up in a home for the elderly for 20 minutes. She was a member of the public who'd come in demanding that my patients be locked in. So I said 'Fair enough' and locked the door. But she was locked in with us. After some 20 minutes she was going berserk, and I wouldn't let her out, and she couldn't even get out of the windows, because they were fitted with burglar-proof locks. Unless you know what it's like to be locked in somewhere you can't glibly say to me 'Well, lock them away. Give them a tranquilliser.'

So far as the average nurse is concerned, the signs and symptoms of dementia are that the patient has no teeth, no hair style, wears anybody's clothes, uses odd slippers that don't fit, has odd socks, never wears braces, and doesn't have a watch. The women don't have handbags and don't wear undergarments. But these aren't the *medical* signs and symptoms of dementia. They're the signs and symptoms of somebody with dementia who happens to be 'in care'. What we're trying to get across is the idea that people suffering from dementia, or who've had a stroke, or who are mentally disabled from any cause, should, if they want, be able to wear make-up, and jewelry, and decent clothes.

I could take you into any psychiatric hospital around here, and what will the men be wearing? They'll be wearing flared trousers and round-collared shirts, for the simple reason that every so often the wives of the nurses say 'It's about time you turned out your wardrobe. You're not going to wear these things any more.' And the nurses say 'Oh, I'm not going to throw them away. It's all good-quality stuff. I'll take them to work with me.' Of course they do, because they realise that Jack and John and George, who've been in hospital all their lives, haven't *got* many clothes. 'So we'll give them these.'

They should be saying 'This man hasn't got any clothes. Let's go out and buy him some new ones. He *deserves* some.' An individual should have his own clothes to wear, and his own shaving tackle, and whatever. The way we dress people in care and in hospital is terrible. If you've dressed smartly all your life, then you want to dress smartly as you grow old. And if you've been scruffy, like me, all your life, you may *want* to look like that.

We try to persuade nurses that they should apply the same standards to their patients as they take for granted for themselves. Take the simple matter of teacups. Nurses don't drink out of patients' cups on the ward. Or if they *do* they feel they have to scour them, send them down to the sterilising unit, boil them in oil, and *then* wash them out again, breathe on them, polish them up, and after all that we use them. But if it's a matter of using that same cup for another patient we just hand it over. If a biscuit falls on the floor it doesn't matter if it's for a patient. You just put it back on the plate again.

I've said to my wife 'If I develop any form of mental illness I'm having a beard, and I don't want it cut. I want a beard down to my knees, and I want that put on my case notes. I don't want *anybody* to shave me, *ever*.' And that's my request, because I've seen so many people being shaved as if the shaver was peeling potatoes, and they have cold water running down their necks – it's a form of torture. Patients are given bed-baths with lukewarm water, and then aren't dried properly.

We don't appreciate what it *feels* like to be on the receiving end of nursing. We don't understand what it's *like* to sit on a commode for half-an-hour, or to sit in the toilet with the door open and have everybody watching you, or for somebody to come up and just grab your handbag and rifle through it to see whether you've got your purse, or whatever, or to have things said about your relatives, or to be told 'You're not *trying*' or 'Look at the mess you've made!'

Nobody will get up and say 'Yes, we *do* apply different standards to these old people.' But we do. We cut corners. 'It doesn't matter if they don't wear knickers' or 'Somebody else's knickers will do for now.' 'She can just wear that cardigan today', even though somebody's brought it in for another patient. 'Don't make any fresh tea. Just heat up the old tea' or 'Just put the milk and sugar in. Don't ask them if they want it. It doesn't matter.' It *does* matter. These little things affect their lives – whether there's salt in the salt pot and pepper in the pepper pot, whether there's sauce on the table, whether they've got knives, forks and spoons, whether the tea's hot, whether they get sugar if they take sugar, or the sugar's left out if they don't.

Cosmic Nursing says the old and the disabled ought to be cared for to very *high* standards, and if you can't meet them you oughtn't to be in the job at all, *or* you ought to be challenging the things that are stopping you.

I often use the attitude of children toward their grandparents to illustrate the way *we* should regard old people. 'When grannies shake hands with you they put 10p in it.' 'They always have clothes that smell of mothballs, and have interesting things in their pockets.' 'They tell you things about your parents that your parents don't want you to know.' To children, grandparents are the kind of people who are always full up when there's only one cake left. Children take a very *positive* view of the old. Nurses tend to take a negative view. 'Oh, they're incontinent. They have bedsores. They've got bad breath. They smell a bit of urine. They can't do this and aren't able to cope with that.' Children have a far more accurate picture of old age than we do.

One of the cruellest deprivations inflicted on the elderly in care is denying them the grandparent rôle. That's why in Cosmic Nursing we always celebrate things like firework night and Christmas – times when your grandpa used to build a bonfire and gran made treacle toffee. The family events should go on, even when you're in hospital.

Relatives come along and say 'Oh, so-and-so's getting married, but I don't think Grandma should really go, because it would be a tiring day for her.' What they really mean is 'It would be embarrassing for us. She'd probably take her teeth out to eat the turkey at the reception.' There's no reason why old people *should* be excluded from occasions like that, or all sorts of other excitements.

The number of people who've written in support of our ideas is phenomenal, and we've now got disciples in various positions throughout the NHS and social services, and a few in the private sector. We can't claim whole wards or whole institutions – just individuals who are isolated little stars dotted around a great black hole. We don't have members, as such, and I'd like to keep it that way, because I think that would make us institutionalised.

As well as writing pamphlets and articles, I do a lot of lecturing. Paul and I used to do skits. I'd dress up as a patient and he'd dress up as a nurse, and we'd do take-offs of the things that happen every day on a ward. Nursing is easy to lampoon, but nurses don't like having their actions and attitudes criticised, and sometimes we'd almost get stoned off the stage. But if you want to change things you've got to be prepared to stick your neck out, and have it knocked off several times. Nurses like to be liked, but we can't afford that luxury.

It's getting to be more than I can manage personally, so at the moment we're making a video and we'll spread the gospel that way.

OPPOSITION

Nobody's ever stood up in public and said we're wrong, and in many ways there isn't actually any argument *against* Cosmic Nursing. The people who don't much like us are those who want to keep nursing very professional, and feel, perhaps, that our ideas somehow threaten the power and authority they want to exercise over their patients.

The usual objection is that our ideals may be fine, but that they can't be put into practice without more staff, more money and more time. To a certain extent I can accept that argument. If you really have *too* few nurses it is sometimes physically impossible to do things like arranging a trip every day.

But I've only *ever* worked in places where the staffing levels were abysmal, and the thing is *how* you work. Most nurses say '*Either* I'm cleaning out a cupboard, *or* I'm talking to residents,' whereas *we* would say 'Go and clean your cupboard and take a resident down to help you, and you can talk while you're doing it. Let him give you a hand.' If you're going to the pharmacy to pick up some tablets, get somebody's hat and coat on and say 'Come with me.' It might not be the best walk in the world, but it's a *walk*. Share out jobs. It's incredible what people are able to do if they're given the chance.

I recently bought a house, and I know nothing about buildings. I thought a damp course was a two-day seminar on incontinence. But we had this very old man with Parkinson's disease who'd been a builder all his life. So on my day off I took him along to have a look. It was a nice 20 minute run in the car, and he had a walk around the house, and gave me his opinion, and I was very grateful. I bought him a pint and a pub lunch on the way back, and he'd enjoyed his day, and he'd been of *use*, and had been practising skills he'd never forgotten. We ought to take old people off the shelf and use them in that way.

It's a matter of approach. You don't have to spend a lot of extra time and money.

A BETTER WAY

By this time I'd decided that there had to be an alternative to long-stay care in hospital, and I wanted to be part of it. A hospital ward is a crazy environment, except for people in need of full-time nursing or medical attention. So I went to work in Part III accommodation. That's the label for the residential homes for the elderly provided by the social services departments of local authorities.

When I made the move they were taking people very similar to the kind you find in long-stay wards, but they were doing the job within a more natural and homely environment. They were accepting mentally-disabled residents because there was nowhere else for them to go – there weren't enough hospital beds available – but I felt it should become official policy, and that homes should be staffed accordingly.

Soon I was asked to take charge of Brookside Home for the Elderly in Ormskirk, where they had some of the best Part III accommodation around. It was a rural area, and there were no long-stay beds locally, so people either had to be taken miles away from home to Winwick Hospital in Warrington, or else they had to come into Brookside. As a result we took a lot of very, very difficult clients, so that to me the job was still to do with nursing, even though you're not employed as a nurse when you work in Part III. Cosmic Nursing was spilling out of the NHS and over into the community.

We set out to treat our people in the way their life history demanded. If you've had a very colourful history, and have been through the Great War, and the depression, and have worked in the cotton mills, and have gone through World War II, and have worked till you're 65, and have been a councillor, or whatever, that should be reflected in the way you're cared for after all that. They should be treated as if they'd *had* a past, and as if they've *got* a present, and as if they've got a *future*. Very rarely do we plan *futures* for people when they grow old.

The average age of the Brookside residents was something like 88, and about a third were over 90. That doesn't mean they haven't got a future. There may be lots of ambitions they haven't fulfilled, and things they'd like to have a go at.

So one of the things Cosmic Nursing achieved at Brookside was to give people the opportunity to do things they either thought they'd never be able to do again or had never been able to do before. It was like an old people's branch of the dangerous sports club. We tried to get away from the myth that old people eat Mint Imperials and like to go to Morecambe for their holidays.

I took a group of men (people had said 'You can't do anything with these people') to a rifle range with the Royal Marine Commandos to let them have a go with live ammunition. It was a great effort to set up, but it was a tremendous success. The marines enjoyed it because for some of them it was the first opportunity they'd had to talk to men who'd actually come under fire. They were due in Northern Ireland in a couple of months, so the younger marines were very interested to hear from people who'd been at Dunkerque or whatever. And these old men, who, three hours before, had been treated as just old people in an old people's home, were being treated by the RMCs as if they were a group more elite than themselves. And this had an effect on the attitude of the staff.

They went to football matches, and not just to *a* football match, but to Old Trafford, to get the atmosphere.

Many elderly people – not all, but some – have led exciting lives, and are used to excitement, and need some in their old age. They need the adrenalin flow. Excitement shouldn't be excluded from old age, whatever disability you may have.

I'd always driven a sports car until recently – until I got married – and I went up to one old man who had quite a severe dementia, and who couldn't actually *speak*, but he'd driven a Morgan all his life, until he was about 79. And I took him out one day, over the moors, in an open-top MG. And the reaction of that man was *incredible*. You could *sense* the adrenalin within him. It was an outing which maybe wouldn't have made a scrap of difference to somebody who'd been used to an ordinary car. But to him...!

Just like those old soldiers being able to get hold of a gun again, and being able to explain to those young soldiers about the old Lee Enfield. They were briefly their young selves again.

I think I can say I've been able to effect *some* change – even if it's only in the lives of a few people.

Chapter 6

A GENTLE PARTING

Dealing with death may well be the main cause of stress among nurses. A study conducted at Bedford General Hospital in 1987 showed that other major stress generators, such as lack of resources, poor staff relationships, difficult old sick people, and low job satisfaction, are regarded by nurses at all levels as far less burdensome than having to cope with dying patients and bereaved relatives. The author of the report, Dr Andrew Guppy, a psychologist at the Cranfield Institute of Technology, suggested that better training might help nurses handle this frequent and bruising experience with less damage to their morale.

Dame Cicely Saunders is the doyenne of an increasing band of doctors and nurses who do not shy away from death but regard the skilled and compassionate care of the terminally ill as a responsibility of prime importance. She was the founder, and is still the mistress, of St Christopher's Hospice in south-east London where some 80 frail old or dying patients have their last days made comfortable and even rewarding.

As a result of her pioneering efforts there is now a growing number of similar hospices. More importantly doctors and nurses at large are being shown how to deal with the physical and emotional pains of the dying.

Dame Cicely is a doctor, but she began her working life as a nurse, which is one good excuse for telling her story here. A second and better excuse is the fact that it is nurses, rather than doctors, who bear the main burden of dealing with death on the ward, and she is the woman who is demonstrating how it should be done.

She has famously said of her patients 'You matter to the last moment of life and we will do all we can, not only to help you die peacefully but to live until you die.'

I'd been up at Oxford for a year when war broke out. I was reading PPE, and I went back for the Michaelmas term of my second year, but over Christmas I decided that Oxford was no place for a girl in wartime. The sister of a friend of mine had gone off to train as a nurse, and it suddenly hit me overnight that that's what I ought to be doing. So I persuaded my father, who *wasn't* very approving, to let me come down from Oxford and train properly, rather than joining the Red Cross or becoming a VAD.

I had a fairly chilly interview at St Thomas' because they weren't that struck on academic people, who they didn't think were going to be very practical. I had to wait a few months before I started, and worked as a VAD in the meantime, but in November 1940 I joined the preliminary training school which was down in the country at Shamley Green in Surrey.

There were around 20 of us. About half were 19-year-olds who were going to do nursing anyway, and the other half were people like me, who wouldn't have been there but for the War.

We did all sorts of things. All our own housework, of course. The food wasn't too bad at that time, though it was nothing special, and it was *freezing* cold. And to my great surprise I found I fitted into a slot for the first time in my life. Having been unpopular at school, and not terribly happy at Oxford, I suddenly knew I was in the right place, and I was thought by the others to be in the right place. I was elected set representative.

Meanwhile St Thomas' had been bombed, so we were sent to Park Prewett, which was a large hospital for the mentally handicapped in Basingstoke, turned into an emergency hospital, with huge wards of 50 or 60 beds filled with soldiers and sailors and so on. It was really hard work. Night duty consisted of 12 on and two off. We had *no* basic equipment. We used paraffin burners to heat the sterilisers. We had no sterile packs, and had to make them up ourselves. So there was an elaborate ritual for *everything* and we were taught pretty much by rote. I still have the book of notes I used when I was revising for my finals – how to nurse a very ill patient, how to do this and that, everything carefully sorted out. Sorting out information and getting it in order has always interested me, and I found exams stimulating, and not an awful great threat, so being a student wasn't hard for me.

Discipline was very strict. I got into terrible trouble at one hospital because I'd agreed to sing for the officers. I used to sing quite a lot, at concerts and so on, and I was asked to sing 'One Fine Day' out of *Madam Butterfly* with the officers at Botleys Park, which was another big mental hospital staffed by Thomas' for the War. Well, I was sent for by the sister tutor and told I was certainly not to do it. 'Sing with the officer patients! You'd find yourself calling them by their Christian names, and how could you then be a nurse – nurse them properly – if you're going to that?' So instead of me going on, one of the officers went on in his wheelchair with his leg sticking out in front of him and sang 'No Nightingales Sing in Botleys Park'.

I used to talk to the men, and had one or two favourites, including one I specialled through a *very* severe illness, and I was actually *encouraged* to do that by the ward sister. Perhaps she was rather enlightened for those days. I got very involved when I was on duty in the children's ward. If a baby died in the night I couldn't bear the porter carrying the body to the mortuary, so I did it myself. I'm not sure if anybody ever found out about *that*!

I wasn't interested in going out with lots of medical students, or staying out late at night. That wasn't my scene. I mean, being asked to sing with the officers was purely because I could *sing*, and for no other reason, and it wasn't particularly in character.

I had some pretty tough sisters who chased me up and down. 'You *can* be good, and you *will* be good. *That's* why I chose you,' one of them said to me. She became a good friend. I don't find discipline particularly difficult. I don't mind working within a structure, so long as I can do what I think I have to do. And I think you can usually find a way.

I really *loved* nursing, and I got interested in cancer at that time, but we didn't have many patients who were dying because they were mostly casualties. I did all right in my finals and got to silver medal standard. They didn't give medals in wartime, but I got an honours certificate.

TWICE BACK TO SCHOOL

I'd suffered from back trouble during my training, and used to have to spend a lot of my off-duty time lying on my bed. It got worse and worse, and by the time I qualified I knew I couldn't carry on nursing.

I was invalided out, and had an operation. It took about six months to settle after that, and then I went back to Oxford to do a wartime degree. I'd been a fairly average student before, and they were expecting my brain would have atrophied, instead of which they found I was *much* better, because I'd learned to work. And I found I was really interested, because I knew what I was doing it for, which was to become a social worker and get back to hospital as fast as I could, because that was my place – the place where I was really happy. I got a distinction in my Oxford degree. It wasn't a proper honours.

I arrived back at Thomas' in the summer of 1947 as what was then called a lady almoner. I didn't start getting involved with dying patients until I'd become a social worker. Then it really hit me, and particularly what it meant to the families.

In the first ward I took over was the man who, as it eventually turned out, became in spirit the founding patient of St Christopher's. He died a few months later in an LCC hospital after having been at home for a while. I'd taken a great interest in his progress, and he left me £500 to do something to remember him by.

After his death I rang up one of the few then existing small homes for the dying – one I'd sent patients to – and asked if I could go along and help as a volunteer. I'd been a very committed Christian since 1945, when I'd said 'What do You want me to do?' But it wasn't until 1948, after my experience with this man, that I knew that the answer was to work with the dying. So I went along to this home, St Luke's, to see if they were 'my kind of people', and whether that was where I was meant to be.

As soon as they found out that I was an SRN they had me working as a sister in the evenings – so there I was, back nursing again! I did that for the next seven years, but after I'd been doing it for two years the surgeon I'd been working for at Thomas' said 'If you're *really* going to do something about the dying you'll have to go and read medicine. If you're going to do something about pain you must do it properly. There's a lot more to be learned. You'll only be frustrated if you don't do it properly, and they won't listen to you.'

Of course, he was right. So then I had to start medicine from the *very* beginning. I got myself into a crammer to try and do first MB, but when my surgeon heard that he marched into the dean's office at St Thomas' and said 'You've got to interview this girl' (or 'this woman' – I was then 33). I'd got a good record of exam performances, and they took me on. So, for the third time, I started at the hospital in a new role.

They'd been taking women for a couple of years by then, and at first I found myself sitting next to a very young girl who was one of the four in our group. I found that terrible. Then I made friends with two or three of the chaps who were a bit older than the others, because they'd been through the Army, and thereafter I had a splendid time and thoroughly enjoyed myself. *And* I kept up my visits to St Luke's.

And I enjoyed working – even slogging through anatomy – just for the sheer joy of getting things on board. I always found chemistry *very* difficult, both in first and second MB, and I needed quite a shove to get through. But I did get through everything, and even got honours in surgery. You see, I knew how to write exams, so it wasn't really such an achievement.

In a way you could say I'm a nurse with extras, or you could say I was tripartite, or you could say I'm just a carer who's had an awful lot of training.

ST JOSEPH'S

I qualified in 1957, and became a houseman, and knew what I intended to do, but had no idea how I was going to do it.

Then my father ran into a professor of pharmacology who'd got some money to do some work on pain, but he didn't have access to patients. He promised me a research fellowship if I could get the patients.

I found that St Joseph's Hospice in Hackney was looking for more doctors. They had about 45 beds for patients with terminal cancer, and provided very dedicated nursing, but with incredibly slender medical support. It was very much custodial care. So I was able to go there, and for the next seven years I worked on developing really *good* pain control.

When I arrived they had no patients' notes, no ward reports, no drug charts – nothing except a DDA book, which you had to have by law for recording all the dangerous drugs given out. We were able to introduce the *regular* giving of morphine and heroin and so on, which I'd seen at St Luke's, and which had been very much the nurses' idea, dating back to the 1930s. The aim was to *prevent* pain, instead of waiting until it occurred and then trying to suppress it.

And that was like waving a wand over the house.

We moved on to working out how to control other distressing symptoms, like nausea and vomiting, and we kept records. I kept patients' notes and drug charts, and the nuns began keeping ward-report books.

Within the next year or two I was able to write a series of articles for the *Nursing Times* about the care of the dying, and, surprisingly enough, they were very well received by the *Lancet*. Then I started being asked to go around lecturing, and by 1963 I'd started travelling to the States.

STARTING A MOVEMENT

I didn't go around lecturing in order to raise money. I went around lecturing to teach. But as a by-product I gradually began to meet people and make contact with trusts, and so on, and as a result I found that it ought to be possible to get the money to *build* a hospice of a kind I knew was needed.

We didn't launch a big national fund-raising campaign. Nobody would have known what I was talking about. Apart from St Joseph's, nobody in this country had even used the word 'hospice'. The King's Fund gave the money for the land in 1963, and then we launched a building fund with just one BBC appeal. The rest was collected by talking to the King's Fund and the Drapers' Company and Nuffield, and so on. We started building St Christopher's in '65 and opened in '67 as the first-ever research and teaching hospice.

We took the academic model of care, research and teaching, and applied it to the care of the dying for the first time. Because of that, and because of the talking and writing I'd done from St Joseph's, we became a catalyst for the hospice movement. I didn't set out to start a movement – but it happened.

With 78 beds we're a little unusual. The average hospice has about 25 beds, and 95 per cent of them just look after cancer patients. We keep eight beds for sufferers from motoneurone disease, and we have 16 in a wing for the frail elderly. There's also a home-care team.

Now that we've been here for 20 years there are quite a few people in the area who've learnt from us, and there are now support teams in most of the local hospitals. As a result the patients who are referred to us are more and more people who've presented difficulties to everybody else. So the physical problems become more complicated, and the family problems become *much* more complicated.

We're tackling difficult situations all the time, but we very much share responsibility and do really work as a multidisciplinary team, with nurses, physiotherapists, social workers, doctors, the chaplain, and a lot of volunteers all involved. The person who picks up a leadership role when it comes to dealing with any particular patient and family might be any member of the team. It moves around the group. The doctors *are* important, but they're not kowtowed to. In a way it's the nurses who tell *us* what to do.

WHAT IT TAKES

Because hospice care is very much a matter of teamwork, you have to be prepared to be open and a part of the community. You have to be interested in people and to feel a concern for the whole family group. You need to be a basic, comfortable, ordinary, resilient being, and you have to be pretty skilful and good at your job. You need to have a good support system of some kind outside. There is a support system inside, but you need other systems outside as well.

I like to hear a nurse applying for a post here say 'We're so busy on our wards that we never have time to talk to the families of dying patients. I want to learn how to talk to families, and I want to know how to talk to patients. I want to learn the skills.'

A lot of our nurses come here for a two-year staff-development programme. In the first six months they work for our certificate, and then they go on to gain experience in the wards, and in management, and in home care. It's quite a sophisticated programme, much helped by the fact that we've got a matron with a lot of flair, and a very, very good senior nurse tutor. But you've got to start with a big interest in people. This means that about half our nurses turn every two years, most of them going back to the NHS, taking what we've taught them under their belts. They go back as ward sisters, perhaps in oncology, or they go into the community as district nurses, and a few go to other hospices. So we have quite a young staff. The nurses in senior posts and the nursing auxiliaries are the ones who tend to stay.

We have some SENs and auxiliaries who are excellent nurses. I would be very sad if auxiliaries ceased to be called nurses. I know they're not in some places. The college doesn't like to *think* of them as being nurses. They argue that a nurse is somebody who's highly trained, so auxiliaries should be called 'aids'. We still call ours '*Nurse* so-and-so'. Our auxiliaries know more about nursing a patient with motoneurone disease than any new staff nurse who arrives, and they *teach* the newcomers how to do it, and that's accepted.

DEATH

In coping with death, efficiency is very comforting. It's not only comforting to the patient and the family, but also to the person who gives it. So we cope with death by being good at pain control, and by being good at the last turning of the patient into the most comfortable position in the bed, and by having sat with the family for a time, or with the patient if the family had to go away. Then you know you've done your best. And we work as a team, so that every patient knows every nurse. We've shared the care, so that when someone dies you're not carrying that sadness on your own.

When a loved person dies – and you never really get used to the desolate crying of that moment, which is different to anything before or after – we always say commendatory prayers, unless the family doesn't want us to. Most families do. That gives something to happen at that moment. There's a card which fits into the nurse's pocket, and she'll usually call up two or three other nurses, so that they can do it together.

On the death of a specially-loved patient, matron will usually try to draft extra help on to the ward, and the chaplain will come in, and so on. Then the full team will go and just sit together over a cup of tea and do their grieving for half-an-hour or more until they're ready to go back and pick up the care of the other patients.

Our people *do* find this draining sometimes, and specially if you have a lot of deaths to deal with, one after the other, and a lot of difficult families.

GOD, AND ALL THAT

A lot of the nurses in the hospice field have got a Christian commitment.

I wrote round to all the hospices a couple of years ago asking 'Do you have a Christian or religious foundation? And if not how do you set out to meet the spiritual needs of your patients?' Roughly half did have a foundation, and some of the others had Christian groups raising money, or said they had one or two Christians on their staff. There were one or two very good answers from nurses in NHS units who were concerned for the *spiritual* rather than the purely religious needs of their patients – a much wider concept. What did emerge was the fact that there are very strong rules about not putting any kind of religious pressure on patients.

This is *not* an evangelistic set-up. But it *is* a set-up in which you hope to create a climate in which people can make their *own* search for meaning, which is very important to them at this stage. We have ward prayers, as quite a lot of hospices would, but some of our patients would rather come to terms with their situation without any words at all.

We are not there to say how it should be done, but we *are* there to answer questions, and wouldn't run away from that. One of the things we've learned is not to say 'Peace! Peace!' where there is no peace.

Because we've been so successful in controlling physical pain and other symptoms, we sometimes tend to think we should be capable of handling spiritual or mental pain in the same way. We can't always do that, and we have to be prepared to just stand by and allow negative feelings to come out.

People move very fast in a crisis, and the fact that patients only spend an average of three weeks in a hospice doesn't mean they're not going to be able to sort out a lifetime's problems in that time. Patients grow in spiritual strength as they lose their physical strength, and you'll see families leaving after a loss more sure of their own resources. A family will find its own strength.

So these are the tremendous rewards of hospice nursing.

Sue Waite is the matron of St Francis Hospice in Havering-atte-Bower, near Romford, and has been in charge since this small institution opened in 1984. Still expanding, St Francis has 20 beds for in-patients, provides day care for a few more, and the staff act as advisers on the management of 50 or 60 people being nursed in their own homes.

Miss Waite acquired her hospice skills at St Christopher's, and is one of the many disciples of Dr Cicely Saunders now spreading the Sydenham gospel abroad. Her mentor describes her as 'Quite young, very plump, a very nice girl, and a very good hospice nurse.'

I *always* wanted to be a nurse. I can't remember ever wanting to do anything else. I think probably the initial thing was the uniform. I really loved the uniform when I was little, and as I grew up and thought seriously about it I became sure *that* was what I wanted to do.

I think all of us in the caring professions feel something about needing to be needed, or needing to be useful, or needing to have some meaning to your life. I'm not sure I was aware of it at the time, but I'm sure that's part of it. And obviously I like people – *most* of the time!

I trained at UCH, starting almost straight from school. At 18 I had no idea of what life was about, but I soon learned, because you're thrown in at the deep end. People *die* on your first ward. Someone grabs you and says 'Help me do this,' with no thought that you've never seen a dead body before, or never seen a man naked before, and don't really know what they look like. You just get on with it. That was about 14 years ago.

I enjoyed the training on the whole. I loved the contacts, and talking to people, but there were parts I didn't enjoy so much. I had to do my children's training at Great Ormond Street, and that made me quite nervous. It was very dramatic, with bells going off everywhere, and I didn't like feeding a baby, and having it start choking, because it had problems in that area.

The other bit I didn't enjoy was neurology and neurosurgery. It was a very stressful ward. It had very ill people in one part who were mostly unconscious, and you had to do all the neuro-observations every quarter-of-an-hour, so you just kept going round and round, and if you stopped you got out of the routine.

One day I got *mad* with the clinical teacher. They used to come round the wards and see how you were getting on, and this woman asked me some really stupid questions while I was trying to cope with six of these unconscious bodies, and she got me totally out of sync. In the end she asked me something, and I said 'I *don't* know, and I don't *care!*' About five minutes later I saw her down at the end of the ward talking to sister. And the remainder of my time on that ward *did not go well*. But the rest I did enjoy.

I wasn't a rebel really. We may have been put upon a bit, but I think I expected that. I spent a lot of my time doing dirty chores. I didn't rebel. I didn't know any better. In fact I quite enjoyed doing the mucky stuff – clearing up and cleaning up – and a lot of it was to do with the actual patient.

The support we got varied. There was a tutor allocated to the trainees and she said 'If you want to talk about anything, come to me.' She was really nice, but when somebody says 'Come and talk to me' that's usually the last person you'd go to. There were some wards where you got very good support, and some where you got absolutely none.

As a fairly junior nurse you'd be left on the ward in the middle of the night, absolutely alone. I think what I did was just not think about it. You just thought 'Well, I've got to get on with it.' If you actually started to think about all the things that *could* go wrong, and *do* go wrong sometimes, you'd just go under.

I remember my first ever night duty. I'd never been up all night before in my life. I was on the postnatal ward, and, of course, at about midnight one of the babies in the nursery started screaming for a feed. And *that's* when I felt that I'd give it all up. I really thought 'I'm never going to do this again.'

That same night the midwife said she was going for a break, so I said 'Fine.' She didn't tell me *where* she was going, and a bit later I had to go to the linen cupboard to get something out. I opened the door, and there was an apparition! It frightened the life out of me. She'd gone to sleep on the floor, and as I opened the door she sat up, and there was this white thing with one of those hospital blankets over her. I'll never forget that night, although they were just stupid little incidents.

I don't think we actually talked about support. It was a new word to me. You just had to get on with it.

TO ST CHRISTOPHER'S

After qualifying I spent six months or so as a staff nurse at UCH and then went to St Christopher's. I went there because I'd read an article in the *Nursing Times* Dame Cicely had written.

We had people dying at UCH, and you did your best, but you always knew, somehow, that there was more you *could* do. You just went in, and turned them over every two hours, and came out. If they asked you anything, you just avoided answering, because nobody had taught you anything different. You weren't encouraged to make relationships with the patients, or to get upset, or to get involved. It just wasn't seen as part of the nurse's life.

And yet it didn't seem right. You were aware that *something* was wrong, but I'd no idea *what* was wrong.

Anyway, I read this article, and I suppose the one thing that particularly appealed to me was the idea that you could not only look after the physical needs, but also the other bits of a person. I was attracted by the idea that you could look after the spiritual needs of a patient, because I've strong beliefs myself, and I could see that there was quite a need for that with people who are dying. I thought 'Well, I'll go and find out how they do it. I might spend a year there. Get the experience and go back.'

I actually stayed for about five years, and I've stayed in hospice work ever since. I started as a staff nurse and eventually worked as a ward sister and then did home care for a while. I went off to another hospice for three months and then went back as the matron's assistant, and then moved to organising home care.

But when I thought about it, what I really wanted to do was to get back to being a ward sister, because that's the high point of nursing. That is *it*. That's real nursing. So I went back to being a ward sister at a hospice in Warwick, and quite enjoyed that time, but I also discovered that having been in a more senior position, you can't really go back, and after 18 months I came here to St Francis, about seven months before we opened.

IN CHARGE

Most of my pressures now come from staff, as opposed to
patients and their relatives, although I do spend some time with
them, particularly now that I'm doing some home-care work. But
normally the stresses are related to management, staff relations,
duty rotas, and that kind of thing. *Some*times it's to do with death
and dying. I think that sometimes what we do in hospices is to react
to the pressures of the work by getting at each other.

When people talk about hospices they seem to feel that they have
to think in terms of an ideal atmosphere, where everything works
beautifully. But there are a lot of occasions when things *don't* go
smoothly, when you *have* trouble controlling some of the difficult
symptoms, and when families *don't* want to have their rifts healed,
and when someone *doesn't* want to talk to you – when someone's
just sick and angry, and that's *it*. If a patient's driving you mad
you may be able to go into the office and shout and scream if you
want to, but sometimes it's easier to take it out on someone else.

We had a problem with the cleaning recently. It wasn't going
very well, and sometimes there was dust under the beds. Obviously
it *was* a problem, but it became an *enormous* problem, leading to
heated arguments. I think the stress of the work gets displaced on
to other things, like dust under the beds, or another member of the
staff, or something like that.

Nurses as a group aren't particularly good at expressing their
feelings, or even *admitting* their feelings. It's trained out of you.
'What are you *doing* nurse?' 'Don't *cry*, nurse!' I'm told it's not
as bad as that now, but it's very difficult to *un*train, and to
say 'It's OK to tell me how you feel. I may *be* your boss,
but that doesn't mean I'm going to think that you're totally
unsuitable if you come and say "I'm really fed up with it
today". We all feel like that sometimes.' So that is quite a
problem – when I see them beginning to get at each other
a bit. It passes.

When I'm interviewing an applicant for a job, the first thing
I look for is whether she's a human being before she's a nurse.
We want the human being part here – relating to other people.
But because you're wanting that, it does mean that nurses pick

up a lot of hurt themselves sometimes, just from seeing other people in distress.

Often nurses want to come into hospice work because they've been disturbed by the bad symptom control they've come across in hospitals or the community. They've seen too many people suffering 'bad deaths', feeling pain, and being violently sick, and so on.

A lot of nurses out there *know* what they should be doing, but haven't got the time to do it, and find in the end that they don't even want to bother. What's the point? We *do* have a larger staff/patient ratio, and we have got more time to do things properly, so that attracts girls who want to be able to care for the whole patient and not just the physical things.

But I have to make sure that they're not just running away from the NHS for what they might imagine to be a soft option. I look to see whether they have some realistic idea of what the job entails. What part of the work do they think will be most difficult for them? A lot say they don't think it will be difficult at all. They think they can come to terms with death, and can cope with the families, and everything will be fine. That worries me, because of *course* it's difficult sometimes. If you've really thought about death you realise it's going to be difficult.

Another question I ask is 'If I gave you £1,000 today, what would you do with it?' They don't understand why I ask that, but the answer gives me some insight into the way a person ticks. There's no right or wrong answer, as I keep telling them.

I don't ask about their faith. This *is* a Christian foundation, and it's very important that there should be people available to talk to patients about such things when they want to, and *if* they want to, but there are a lot of the nurses who would get someone else to do that. Quite a number of the nurses here do have some particular religious belief, but quite a number don't. I think I'd worry if I found myself with a hospice full of nurses who were *all* unbelievers, but I don't think I could cope with one *full* of committed Christians. They can be a bit overpowering, sometimes.

I firmly believe in God, and count myself to be a committed Christian, but some of the others I've met are pretty obnoxious. People are people, whatever their beliefs. I've met some excellent nurses who are agnostic, and maybe atheist, and I've met some terrible ones who are professing Christians. Christianity doesn't make you perfect, and it's not a requirement for service here.

We don't have any male nurses at the moment, although we have had, and it helps. This hospice, like, I suppose, a lot of hospices, is a matriarchal society. There are *so* many women. It can be nauseating, and it adds a bit of normality to have a few men around. It gives you a different perspective – a different way of looking at things – and certainly some of the male patients appreciate it. Male nurses have got as much to give as female nurses. A man is not a woman and a woman is not a man. We *are* different, and we *do* see things in different ways, sometimes. It does help men to be able to talk to men sometimes.

DOCTORS

I have very little faith in doctors. You tend to start off with the belief that the members of the medical profession are almost gods. You can't help it. And then, when you look at what goes on, the pendulum swings completely the other way, and you think 'My God! What a shower!'

Sometimes doctors do make themselves out to be gods, and they make their decisions without a proper consideration for all the circumstances of their patients. If they wanted to give me a treatment or some operation I didn't want, I'd say so. But I *wouldn't* have done. My mother would think 'If the doctor says you need this, then you need it, and no questions asked.' You don't say 'What are you trying to do?' or 'What's it for?' or 'What are the side effects?' You don't question what the doctor says. You just *do* it.

Patients do come here sometimes who've had unnecessary treatment, and their doctors know that – that it's not going to improve that patient's chances of survival – but they go on doing it. I think that's because a lot of doctors see death as a failure. I think a lot of people go into doctoring because they *want* to be gods, and they want to have power, and they want to make things better for people. They want to be needed and to prove themselves worthwhile.

And, of course, they often achieve this. But then if someone dies, and your reason for being is to make people better, then you *do* feel a failure. I think a good many doctors try to avoid thinking about death, and have never even thought about their own death. They can't cope. They pass by the end of a dying person's bed without saying anything. Everybody stops talking to these people, and they *know* something's up.

The teaching needs to be improved, and I think nurse training *is* improving. When we hold our seminars here we get a lot of community and hospital nurses coming – and very few doctors.

I don't really want to doctor-bash, but I do get a bit cross and despairing when they don't do quite simple things in the way they should. If someone's got bone pain, then you give them something for bone pain, which seems to me *extremely* simple, and it's been bandied about for years. Yet doctors still just don't do it, and those patients are suffering excruciating pain. They've had no training in terminal care – how to deal with the physical symptoms, and how to look after the dying *person*. We've still got a long way to go in educating people.

But you have to do it so gently. Unfortunately people see it as a threat. If you say 'How about doing it *this* way?' when they've been doing it some other way for years, and think they've been doing it properly, it hurts their pride – specially with doctors.

Obviously, they're all different. Some of the younger ones I came across during my training were obviously extremely nervous, and didn't really know what the hell they were doing. But they were all right.

I've met some fairly strong consultants who knew exactly how they expected things to be done, and that was *that*. 'Stand respectfully by the bed.' 'Have the patient lying neatly at attention as the consultant comes round.'

Some doctors treat nurses as fellow professionals, but there are quite a lot who don't and regard us as their handmaidens – as somebody to clear up afterwards when they leave their dirty syringes and needles lying around. Sometimes we bring it on ourselves, because we won't stand up to the medical profession, and just *take* it. Nurses in general *are* becoming more vocal, and becoming stronger, and sticking up for themselves.

But there's an awful long tradition to be overcome of just 'taking it all'.

I've heard more stories about nurses being put upon than I've experienced myself. I don't stand for any nonsense. Having said all that, I'll admit to having got on with doctors very well – on the whole.

FACING UP TO DEATH

I've accused doctors of shying away from death, but nurses do it too.

There's a family around here with a dying child at home, and one of the community nurses had gone in. It was her first visit, and she was new to the job, but she was well aware of the fact that the mother had been looking after this kid at home for a long while, and when the mother said 'Hallo, nurse,' she said 'Don't call me nurse. Call me sister.' The mother's a super woman, and was very graphic in her description of the scene, and that said to me that the nurse wasn't coping with the stress of handling an 11-year-old boy who was dying. She was hiding behind her professional role.

It *is* difficult. We don't *know* what to do, and we want to put a plaster on it. We want to stop someone crying, and say 'There, there! It'll be all right!'

But you can't do that with death. It is *painful*, it is *parting*, it is *leaving* things, it is unfulfilled ambitions, there is *pain* there – and you can't put a plaster over it. So you run away from it. You make another cup of tea.

In some ways you do get used to patients dying. There are the routine things to be done. There are the relatives to be cared for. And it's not all affecting you, all the time, because I suppose if it did you wouldn't survive. In fact it probably *is* affecting you. You're just not aware of it.

One of our coping mechanisms is to make little jokes. I sometimes listen to the jokes made by the staff, and by myself, and think 'Gosh! If somebody who didn't work in a hospice heard that they'd think we were absolutely terrible.' We laugh about things we've heard from the mortuary. It's just a coping mechanism.

I suppose you don't ever get used to it, but you do, in a way, sail through a number of deaths without any obvious reaction. But every now and again somebody really gets to you. I think if deaths didn't *ever* affect you, that would be quite frightening.

PROSPECTS

I don't think I'd want to stay in hospice work for the rest of my working life. I've quite a few years to go yet, and I don't *know* what I want to do. Where do you go after being matron of a hospice?

When I was interviewed for this job they said 'How long do you see yourself staying?' I said 'Between five and ten years.' I'm not even at five yet, but I'm beginning to wonder what I'll do next.

At the moment we're very much in the expansion stage, so I don't feel I'm in a rut. We've got the in-patient unit going, and the home-care unit going, but we're expanding our day care, and want to expand our education role, so there's a lot to be done, and while there *is* a lot to be done, I'm happy doing it.

I'm not sure I want to go back into the NHS. I don't want to go back into that rat race. I don't want to go back into a situation where you don't have time to do things properly. But maybe I shall, just to teach them how it should be done.

Perhaps I'll go into counselling. I'm actually doing a counselling course at the moment, because it's the trendy thing to do.

So long as it's to do with people. OK, I've got a mortgage and a car and the bank manager keeps writing me nasty letters and I do worry about money.

But, in the end, it's people that matter.

Chapter 7

PRISON

Michael Jenkins is a senior hospital officer at Pentonville Prison. He provides prime proof of the fact that a nurse is a nurse, is a nurse, whatever the setting.

When I left school I became a civil servant, working for the DHSS, but at that time we were so poorly paid that I could barely exist. The prison service offered more money. It was as simple as that.

I did almost a couple of years as a discipline officer and then transferred. Looking back it's difficult to know exactly why. I just decided that being a discipline officer wasn't what I wanted to do for the next 30 years. You can become a PE instructor, or a works officer, or go into catering. There are various specialisations within the job. But I decided that working in the hospital, with the variety of experiences that entails, would be something I could do for 'X' years to come.

I'd only gone into the prison service to earn more money, and to get a free house, and there was nothing altruistic about it, but as soon as I started the hospital training I knew that that was what I wanted to do.

We did a three-month course in those days in our own school of nursing. It's six months now. But within that time you get through about the same amount of theoretical work as you get during the first 18 months of SRN training, and we also did about four weeks practical – two weeks general nursing in an NHS hospital, and two weeks in psychiatry.

Then you start as a hospital officer (HO) on 12 months probation. It's very similar to being an SEN, but at times you're expected to shoulder rather more responsibility. In a large prison like this we have doctors available from nine to five, but outside those hours you have to take your own decisions regarding the initial assessment of a patient, and so on. In a small establishment you might only have a GP coming in once a day, and in an emergency you'd be expected to decide what to do, and what immediate treatment might be needed, even as an HO, and somebody who's unqualified in the eyes of the rest of the nursing world.

A newly-appointed HO has done more hours in school than a student nurse in the NHS, and has the head knowledge, perhaps, but what you lack is confidence and experience, and I'd say it takes two or three years to gain that to the extent that you feel fully comfortable in the job. I know the department would like to extend the training period still further, but under the present financial constraints, six months is all the Home Office will allow.

MAKING A PROPER JOB OF IT

I did a couple of years as an HO, and then I decided to take special leave to train as an SRN, so for the next three years I existed on the pay of a student nurse. I went to the North Middlesex, and had a thoroughly good time. I enjoyed every single area I was in. I had a good background in basic nursing care, so things like taking temperatures and blood pressures and making beds, and even the drugs, weren't new to me.

There were just two of us men among all the women, but that didn't worry me a bit. To a certain extent I think I had it easier *because* I was a male, and also because I was older, and married. I think it meant I wasn't given the runaround so much as some of my colleagues! The biggest problem I had initially was having to remember that I couldn't make my own decisions about nursing care in the way I'd been used to doing. I had to refer to somebody else.

I was well accepted by the other nurses, and by the patients. I think patients do still find the idea of a male nurse a bit unusual. A male charge nurse is accepted, because he obviously *is* in charge, but a male student still seems a bit strange to people, and some had a mental block about addressing me as 'Nurse'. I used to get them to call me by my first name, just because it made them feel more comfortable. I don't care *what* people call me.

There was no trouble with the female patients. The school had only recently been visited by the General Nursing Council, as it then was, and had been told to get itself into the 20th century in the matter of allocating posts to male nurses, and they then went over the top the other way, so that I spent 60–70 per cent of my ward training on the female side. I think, again, the fact that I was married and that much older helped, so that perhaps they saw me as a husband who *knew* about women.

While I was doing my obstetrics I had an Asian lady who'd come in for a late booking. It happened to be my one week that you do as a student in the booking clinic. She was the first lady I'd ever interviewed on my own, and I think the midwives had set me up with her as a joke, because she didn't speak any English. She did bring her sister along to translate, but the sister didn't speak much more English than I spoke whatever language they were talking. So I had a very interesting three hours struggling through an interview that should have lasted half-an-hour, all on my own, except that the midwife came in to do the actual examination.

Two weeks later I was on the labour ward and this same Muslim lady was admitted – in labour. There was a big note on her records saying that because of her religious convictions she refused to be seen by any male doctor, whatever happened. But since I'd looked after her originally I asked the sister in charge whether I could follow this lady through the course of her delivery, assuming she was willing. Sister said 'Well...yes. But in view of this note you'll have to play it by ear.'

In the event the lady would *not* let me leave. I prepared her, and undressed her, and took the initial observations, and put the foetal monitor on, and when the time came to go into the delivery room she dismissed her sister, but would *not* let me leave. I stayed for the delivery, and then admitted her up to the ward. It was a smashing experience for me, and she was happy. I don't think my gender entered into it. I was just a friendly face she *knew*. I think that was more important than gender. The following day I got a big box of chocolates and a card addressed to 'Mr Michael'. That caused a bit of derision.

But I had no problems with the women at all. Obviously you use some discretion with the younger ladies – even the older ones. If ever they'd said they were embarrassed, or I'd *felt* they were, I'd have changed my approach, or perhaps have called someone else. But it never happened.

All nurses will say that patients get attached to you. I had three boys at the time, and often, when the hospital shop came round, someone would buy three bars of chocolate, and whisper 'Take these home to the children.' I'd bring in pictures of the children to show them, and that established a relationship. I was another human being, and not just an anonymous nurse in a white coat.

I had a super time.

BACK TO PRISON

As soon as I'd qualified I came back to my HO job – to the same rank.

On the female side of the prison service they've always employed plenty of qualified nurses, but on the male side the tradition has been to employ prison officers who've done the HO training.

I was more experienced by now, of course, and I was looked upon and used in that way. I was consulted about things other people found difficult, while getting on with my own job. But the main thing that changed was my relationship with the doctors. I was more professionally accepted, and my opinions were given more weight.

The other thing that happened was that I went before a promotion board a few months ago and got upgraded to senior hospital office at my first attempt. I think I'd have been promoted eventually, anyway, but I expect the fact that I'd applied myself to doing something extra helped to speed things up. But there's no question of having to be an SRN in order to get promotion.

There are three grades of nursing staff here. We have two principal officers (POs), three SNOs, and should have 16 HOs. We've actually got ten. Today there should be one PO on duty, and 14 others. In fact there's one PO and *six* others. That's not unusual. Everybody's overworked. It's just as bad as the NHS. One of the POs is a registered mental nurse. Two of the HOs are SRNs, and one's an SEN, and there's myself. So there are five of us with nursing qualifications. The rest have just done the HO course.

Actually, the mix we've got at the moment works very well because there's always at least one professionally-qualified staff member around, so although the others are expected to make their own decisions, if they're faced with a situation beyond their experience or capability, there's someone to go to for advice.

There's a full-time senior medical officer, and two full-time MOs, plus a local GP who does the prison sick parade four days a week, and we have various visiting consultants.

We've just started employing female agency nurses, who are nothing to do with the prison service. The only stipulation is that they should be cleared by the Criminal Records Office before they're allowed through the gates. That's the nature of the establishment.

We do have one female HO, who was a discipline officer at Holloway, and we'll be getting another one. This is new.

We don't have any discipline staff within the hospital. We're a separate entity.

We're catering for the nursing needs of 1,200 inmates, and we get the whole range of illnesses to treat. We get a large proportion of mentally ill, and a lot of drug addicts and alcoholics, and a few subnormals. Prisoners, statistically, are not very well. All the same, at any one time only 45 or 50 are ill enough to be in hospital.

We've got 52 beds, of which 17, in theory, are for psychiatric patients. There's a 12–bed ward, and a six-bed ward, and the rest are single rooms. In reality the majority of our single medical rooms are used for overspill psychiatric patients.

We keep the more fractious and troublesome of our psychiatric patients on the psychiatric landing, but the better ones – those well enough to conform to a reasonable regime – go on the medical landing in a single room. One or two, suffering from some exogenous depression, we'll nurse in one of the wards, because very often company helps. We have some very difficult psychiatric patients. They take up half our time.

On the medical side we deal with everything apart from pre- and post-op care. We don't have a theatre. Wormwood Scrubs, Parkhurst and Liverpool have full surgical units. We don't.

We're separate, and we *stay* separate, from the main prison. We stay separate from the main staff because we want to make the point that our professional role is *caring* for our patients. So far as 95 per cent of them are concerned, we'll have no idea of what their sentences are, or what crime they've committed, or why they're on remand. Most of us do that deliberately. We'll only find out if their offence has a real relationship to their nursing needs – if they're child molesters, for example, and they're in here for assessment. Then their crime becomes relevant to their treatment. But only then would we find out.

SICK PARADES

Within the main prison every inmate has a right to report sick at any time, and they have a right to see a doctor within 24 hours.

There's a sick parade held there every morning, just as there is in the armed services, and around nine-o-clock they come down to see the doctor. The parade's manned by an SNO and two HOs. The doctor prescribes, and then the SNO passes on the instruction to one of the HOs, who will carry out the treatment, be it medication, or a dressing, or whatever.

There are three treatment times as well, first thing in the morning, at lunchtime, and at teatime, when prisoners on the sick list are seen, and are given whatever medicines they've been prescribed. That's in addition to the sick parade. So there's an opportunity to be seen up to four times daily by a hospital officer. And any time if anybody tells the discipline staff that they want to go what we call 'special sick', out of normal time, they must be seen by an HO as soon as possible.

All prisoners have immediate access to medical care. We have about 250 medicines handed out within the main prison each day. They vary right through, from antibiotics, to common cold cures, and psychotropic drugs. Actually we use psychotropics very sparingly. This is partly because over the past four or five years we've become acutely aware of being accused by the popular press of using them as a 'liquid cosh'. But, in fact, it's never been the policy to use much in the way of tranquillisers and so on here, and the same patients would receive far more if they were being treated in a mental hospital. This is a secure environment, and people don't have the freedom and latitude they would have in an open psychiatric ward outside, so we don't *need* to medicate them just to maintain control.

We've had patients come here from other establishments who have been over-medicated, and we'll stop their drugs initially, for three or four days, unless they're *very* agitated, just to allow them to have a proper medical and nursing assessment. Then, even if they do go back on the tablets, we'll only use fairly small doses. It's nice to see somebody getting much better when that happens.

All my staff are authorised to dispense ordinary household remedies, like paracetamol, or magnesium trisilicate for an upset stomach, without the patient having to see a doctor. But if any inmate *insists* on seeing the doctor, that's his right.

ON REMAND

We have a fairly quick turnover of patients because of the nature of their sentences. There are no long-term prisoners. The ones who tend to stay with us longest are those on remand. They can be waiting for trial for anything up to two years. It's frightening. It would upset *me* to be in limbo for that length of time, and it doesn't make life any easier for us in our nursing role, because you've got somebody who's mentally distraught before you start.

A proportion won't be given a custodial sentence in the end, and if they are convicted, and have already served 12 months in custody, they *must* be given a sentence of *more* than 18 months, otherwise they'd have served their time already, because one-third remission is automatic. And if somebody's served two years on remand, which is not impossible, and is given less than a three-year sentence, he'd already have served *more* than his time. So whatever happens, don't have your case heard at Snaresbrook. That's the two-year wait. All the inner London courts are over 12 months.

We also have detainees and deportees and prisoners in for contempt of court. Every prisoner sentenced for contempt is seen by us and medically assessed by one of the doctors. A letter has to be sent to the Official Solicitor, because someone may well have been in contempt because of mental illness rather than any deliberate defiance.

DRUNKS AND ADDICTS

We have ten or 12 drunks and five or six drug addicts admitted to the prison every *night*, and a proportion of them will end up here. The rest we can manage to treat within the main prison. But they're all seen and monitored over that first critical period of withdrawal, which lasts ten to 14 days. We reckon that's a speciality of ours, because we see so many of them.

The general mortality rate for people developing DTs is around 10 per cent, but we haven't lost a single patient from that cause within living memory, and we're quite proud of that. That's because we recognise the precursors very quickly and start treatment right away.

We've always treated drug addicts symptomatically, and have never used replacement therapy. We don't give Physeptone as a heroin substitute. Instead we give whatever sedatives and anti-emetics and anticonvulsants may be needed to keep the patient stable. But withdrawal symptoms are closely related to the treatment you provide. The more treatment somebody thinks he can get out of the system, the worse he claims and maybe feels himself to be. It's a psychological thing. They just want *some* kind of drug.

Curiously enough, severe withdrawal symptoms are very much a thing of the past. In the late '70s we used to see quite severe *physiological* reactions, which required large doses of anti-emetics and anticonvulsants for their control. I haven't seen that for three or four years, and yet we're getting the same number coming in who *claim* to be drug addicts, and who say they're fixing, mainlining, smoking, or whatever, just as much as before. They're every bit as dependent psychologically as they always have been, but physiologically the problems are far less. It can only be that the quality of the drugs they're using in the streets now has gone down. The drugs are being cut. People aren't taking nearly so much of the active drug as they think they are.

We don't see the opium eaters any more. They used to come in with serious gastrointestinal problems, but now we have opium smokers instead, especially among the Chinese. Their treatment is sometimes made more difficult by the existence of a certain amount of ethnic resentment. We're very careful to make sure that no overt racial discrimination is allowed to happen here, but often patients belonging to other ethnic groups seem to believe that because we're Anglo-Saxon we're out to harm them medically. They think we'll not only put them in prison and lock them up, but try to poison them as well.

EXPERT ATTENTION – FAST

We see around 100 inmates on the morning sick parade, so the amount of consultation each gets is pretty minimal. For anything that can't be dealt with there and then the prisoner's put on 'call-up', which means he attends as an out-patient in the hospital. The doctor will probably see half-a-dozen every morning, and half-a-dozen in the afternoon, and can spend as much time with each as might be needed.

There's a VD clinic on two half-days a week, run by a visiting consultant from the Royal Free. There's a dentist for three full days a week, and an optician comes for half-a-day.

Three of the HOs have been away to qualify as radiological technicians, so we take our own X-rays, but a consultant radiologist comes in to read them once a week, and at other times when needed. A consultant chest physician comes in on one or two days a week, and a consultant psychiatrist is here for two or three days. The psychiatrist is a workaholic, and helps a lot in finding prisoners places in mental hospitals. He's got influence.

That's a real problem throughout the prison service, because we've always got mentally ill patients who really ought to be in psychiatric hospitals. It's a matter of finding someone willing to take them. Our own psychiatrist and a psychiatrist from the catchment area concerned may both agree that a patient ought to be 'sectioned' under the Act – ought to be made a compulsory patient in a mental hospital. But then we'll get a deputation of nurses coming to see him, and 60 per cent of the time they'll veto having the patient on their ward, either claiming that the man's mentally fit, or isn't treatable.

I can understand their reluctance to accept difficult customers. We might find them easier to deal with because they're within a secure, defined environment. Nevertheless, we sometimes view their decision with a certain amount of suspicion.

That problem apart, our patients do see specialists very quickly. They'll get an appointment to see an orthopaedic surgeon, for example, within two or three weeks, which is far faster than I could arrange for my own family. There's often a waiting list of a year or more.

Unfortunately we had an inmate die here a couple of months ago. He was a young man who had a rare combination of thyrotoxicosis *and* myasthenia gravis. He had a myasthenic crisis, and we resuscitated him, but he died later in the day in casualty at the Whittington from cardiac arrest. In his summing up the coroner said he probably wouldn't even have been *diagnosed* as a myasthenic if he'd been going to his GP.

Then there was a lad I took to the Whittington only the other day. He'd been treated for asthma for six months by his GP because he was wheezy. He came into the prison one night and we saw him next morning. He had pitting oedema up to the groin. He was wheezy. He had a systolic murmur even *I* could hear. When we took a proper history we found he'd been suffering from rheumatic heart disease since the age of 14. He was in heart failure, and yet he'd been given a Ventolin inhaler and sent on his way. I don't suppose the GP ever even took the poor man's shirt off.

They kept him in, and he's been decategorised, which means he has open prison status, and is on trust while he's there. He's only doing a short term. So he's now getting the medical treatment he requires, which he wouldn't have done if he'd carried on outside. He's still serving his sentence, but is going to be in hospital for pretty well all the time, *and* is being treated for something that was killing him.

You can berate the GP for missing the diagnosis, while we saw what was wrong, but that's basically because we have a little more time.

A LARGER ROLE

The Home Office is now encouraging qualified nurses to apply for direct entry as hospital officers. They still have to do six months' prison training to start with because of our dual role.

I've said we keep ourselves separate from the discipline staff, but we're none the less responsible for security within the hospital, and we have to be familiar with all the rules and regulations, and prisoners' entitlements in the matter of visits and letters and so on. We wear the same uniform as discipline staff, except that we have an H on the lapel or shoulder strap. I wear a white coat on the landing.

I hope getting more qualified nurses in, and eventually, perhaps, having *all* qualified staff, will enhance the status of the service in the eyes of the profession as a whole, as well as improving the care we can give our patients, although I have to say that one of the best nurses I've ever worked with was not professionally qualified. He retired a year go. I've never worked with a better nurse at *any* grade. And we have some excellent HOs who are highly skilled at nursing people well within our peculiar environment.

The pay's good. In the NHS the best I could have hoped to achieve at this stage is to have become a charge nurse, which is a similar grade to the one I'm in now, but the pay's appalling, whereas my pay for this year will be something over £19,000 – more than double.

In spite of that we do find it difficult to get nurses to come in. It does take.a peculiar kind of person to work within this environment. I don't mean that in any derogatory sense, but we are dealing with people who have been excluded from the rest of society.

You can't say 'Get your wife to bring in a packet of biscuits tomorrow,' or 'Ring up your girlfriend and ask her to buy a postal order for the pools.' They do *not* have free access to the outside world. They do *not* have free access to a telephone. They have a visit for half-an-hour *once* a fortnight, and the rest of the time you must be their entire support. You are caring for their every need. We arrange visits for them. We end up being their father confessors, and their mothers, and the brothers they never had, all rolled into one, and they very much see us as that.

Also, you're locking them in. All right – we're caring for them as patients, but none the less at the end of the day we're locking the door and making sure they don't run away, and it's not always easy to accept that you have that custodial role as well. So we do have a dual role, and we have an enhanced role.

We have far more responsibility than you'd have on an NHS ward. We're consulted rather than instructed by the medical staff. We're expected to reason things out for ourselves. Whereas nurses in the NHS are fighting to be considered as individual practitioners, we *accept* that, and *expect* that of our staff. I expect them to make decisions. I might reason with them, or criticise them afterwards, but I don't expect them to come running to me with every problem, unless they're out of their depth and confused. We aim to make the best use of every skill each officer has, regardless of paper qualifications.

PROSPECTS

I expect I'll stay in the service until I retire. Apart from anything else I couldn't afford to leave.

I started working for a diploma in nursing, paid for by the department, which is a three-year day-release course, but my wife unexpectedly became pregnant again, and the combination of a new baby and the extra work became too much, so I had to drop out. There's quite a lot of work involved.

I shall have another go at the start of the new academic year, either going back to the diploma or starting something else, because I find nursing fascinating, both academically and practically, and I think we've got room in this service for people who are committed to professional nursing standards.

It's probably easier for us to go on courses of that nature than it would be in the NHS, because, although we're tight for money, we're not quite as tight as some of the health authorities.

The whole prison service is undergoing a great change. The routine has gone on for many years, mostly working very well on our side, although we have been rather old-fashioned, often making do with Victorian facilities, and under-exploiting the capabilities of the staff because of a lack of resources. But recently we've had an influx of qualified staff from the NHS, bringing in new ideas, and we're getting more and more updated with our equipment and techniques.

There are still a lot of things that could be improved, but the civil service, like any large organisation, does move slowly. All the same, things *have* changed over the last few years, sometimes at my insistence. You can see you've actually accomplished something, albeit not quite as quickly as you'd like. But you can't bring about change from the outside. That's got to be done from the inside.

Having said that I believe our patients get care equal to the best on offer within the NHS, and I'm unashamedly enthusiastic about what we're doing.

I enjoy it. I'm frustrated on occasions. None the less, I enjoy it thoroughly.

Chapter 8

GOING ABROAD

There are all sorts of reasons for going abroad to nurse. It may be to escape. It may be to adventure (which could be the same thing). It may be to discover what other kinds of people are like, or, in a missionary spirit, to attempt to make other kinds of people more like one's self. Or it may be just to earn a bit more money. Nobody opting to serve as a nurse in a third world country under the auspices of Voluntary Service Overseas would do so for the last of these motives, because the rule is that volunteers have to make do on whatever the going rate for the job may be in the place where the work is done.

Lilian Brodbin had worked in the NHS for 20 years before she decided to 'go abroad' with VSO, and 'loved every minute of it'. But, while devoted to the concept of the NHS, she didn't even consider rejoining the service when she returned to the UK after her time away. Poor staffing levels and an increasing bureaucratic interference with the day-to-day activities of the workers at the sharp end of the game had, to her, reduced job satisfaction to an unacceptably low level. So, when I spoke to her, she was the matron of a ritzy private nursing home in Bournemouth. A bit of a change from the conditions she'd experienced, and enjoyed, in Liberia, not many months before.

110

She's a 'gin-and-tonic' woman of the nicest and most valuable kind.

I became a nurse for a really silly reason. I was a nursery nurse at around the time of Suez, and I thought 'Well, what could I do if there was a war?' And I thought 'I could be a nurse, and *that* would be useful.' And that's why I did it.

I went through the lot in the NHS, all the departments in various hospitals – night sister, everything – but in the end I applied to VSO for purely selfish reasons. I wanted to see other cultures. I knew there was *something* beyond the street outside the hospital.

They told me there wasn't much need for nurses unless they had some speciality. Maybe they were trying to put me off. Maybe they thought that at my age I needed putting off. But they didn't succeed, because I went off and did my midwifery training. And when I went back with that they took me on.

I was sent out to Liberia, together with another girl, Ada, who was a nursing manager, six or seven years older than me. We were the first two VSOs in the country, but later we were joined by another VSO in the educational field, who was ten or 12 years older still, so we were quite a geriatric group. Most volunteers are in their 20s or 30s, but I think they'll take you up to 65. Age isn't a determining factor, which is rather nice.

Ada and I had been given the job of organising primary health care in some of the villages. At first I was very scared, because although that was what I wanted to do – get to work in the villages – and although I was supposed to be the visiting expert, I actually knew nothing about it. It was a matter of learning the job as you went along, without any guidance at all, and I was quite surprised at how quickly you picked it up. There was nobody there who could give you any advice, or support, or anything. I had my little bible, *Where There Is No Doctor*, and got by with that.

I looked after the training side, and Ada managed the organisation and finances. I also had a Liberian counterpart called Grace, who was excellent. She'd trained as a midwife. It's VSO policy that you have a national working alongside you who can take over and carry on when you leave.

We had a sponsor, Plan International, which is an American-based charity, and they paid our salaries. The Liberian government was the other half of what was meant to be an equal partnership. The government was supposed to provide transport and fuel and so on, but *didn't*. It happens in all the third world countries, and particularly Liberia, which is now bankrupt. We never had a penny from them. They did provide Grace, and space for an office in a building attached to the hospital in the township where we were based.

Unfortunately Plan International felt very strongly that they should only provide half the needs of the project, and in theory they were right, because the idea was to encourage the Liberians to stand on their own feet, against the time when we should leave, but it didn't help us at *all*, and when we arrived we had *nothing*. Ada had brought some pencils with her, and we were cutting them into *thirds*. It was as bad as that. But Plan provided some drugs, which we sold, and with that income, and a bit of money sent out by friends, we got going.

THE SCENE

We were working over brush and scrubland, with a little bit of virgin forest, and communications were virtually non-existent. Fortunately we got hold of a four-wheel-drive vehicle provided by UNICEF, otherwise we'd have been scuppered. There were no wild animals – no nasties – because they'd all been hunted out. But there were masses of snakes. We were all terrified of the snakes.

The idea was to create and train village health workers, and to show the traditional birth attendants how to do a rather better job. These were the women who delivered babies in the villages. They had no kind of training. They just followed tribal customs.

There hadn't been any such thing as a village health worker. This was a new concept. The villagers relied on the medicine man, and the bone doctor, and the black beggar. Black beggars were the itinerants who used to go round giving injections, mostly of antibiotics, which were very freely available, or they'd give out one or two antibiotic tablets, and that was it. No question of a complete course. You could go into the market and buy a tablet or two of an antibiotic, and they'd take them for the most ridiculous things, like a headache or a common cold. The misuse of antibiotics was phenomenal.

So there were no trained health workers in the villages, and the traditional birth attendants (TBAs) were behaving in the most alarming fashion. They'd put mud or cow dung on the cut end of the birth cord, which was bad enough, but the worst of their habits was the beating of a woman in prolonged labour. The theory was that a difficult labour meant that a woman had been unfaithful to her husband, so that she had to be punished before labour could progress. And they were beaten very, very severely. We had a lot of women with dislocated hips and broken thighs. We did manage to persuade them that this was *not* a good idea, which was one of our greatest achievements.

The mothers weren't too good at breastfeeding. They were better up north, but the nearer you were to Monrovia, the more inclined they were to use the bottle, because that's what all the élite city people did. But the villagers didn't know how to handle artificial feeding properly, and it caused the most awful malnutrition. They also thought their milk was ruined if they went back with their husbands, and that if their husbands wanted them back they had to stop breastfeeding. And they thought colostrum was a bad thing – 'spoilt milk' – so they got rid of that and didn't start feeding until they were on to the 'good milk'.

When it came to weaning they'd give the babies 'fru-fru', which is just a starchy material looking like wallpaper paste, and with about the same nutritional value, I suspect. Some women would feed their babies just on that up to about a year, so you ended up with a highly malnourished child.

If the baby wouldn't eat they'd go in for a kind of forced feeding. They had a word for it. They'd lie the infant on the lap and just *shove* food and water down its throat, and the child would be screaming its head off. That caused a lot of pneumonia and deaths. They didn't think it was their fault, of course. If the baby died, that was from some other cause. They'd done their best.

Ada drew up this marvellous statistical thing. I can't remember the figures offhand, but I know we had one of the highest infant mortality rates of any third world country, mostly because of diarrhoea and malnutrition.

Malaria was one of the commonest diseases. VD was rampant. So was gastroenteritis, because of contaminated water. We had a report of just one AIDS case over the radio while I was there, but were told that 'Nobody need worry, since the patient had died.' I thought that was lovely. I think there were probably a lot more who weren't being diagnosed. Malnutrition was widespread.

In fact there was plenty of good food available – everything you could possibly want. Lots of cassava – the roots are just starch, but the leaves are very strong in nutrients. And every village had hundreds of citrus trees, but they wouldn't eat the fruits at all. The problem was that they grew everything to *sell*, and just ate dried rice themselves. I'm not sure who actually bought the stuff, apart from white people like me.

They did have latrines in the villages, but most of them were locked up, and were only for VIPs, so they weren't used. Anyway, some of them were so badly constructed that when you went in you were hit by a swarm of flies, so they were more of a hazard than a benefit. It was safer to go in the bush.

Worms were very prevalent – hookworms and tapeworms. They used to save them in little bottles for us to inspect every time we went round. We'd treat them, and the worms would come out, and that was something you could actually *see*. That was a great success.

HOSPITALS

The hospital scene out there was absolutely appalling. We had this office attached to a government hospital. The mattresses were filthy and had great big holes in them. People were being asked to bring in their own mattresses. There was no water in the hospital at all. Can you imagine a hospital without *water*? And it goes without saying that there was no electricity.

Most of the time they were out of drugs, and had no anaesthetics, but it happened that, just as we arrived, so did 13 Chinese doctors, and they'd decided to keep all 13 of them in just this one hospital. We had acupuncture going like mad, although they were western-trained and had among them anaesthetists and various other specialists. They'd brought their own drugs, which they'd reckoned would last a year, but they went in six months, because *everybody*, from the whole of Liberia, started turning up. Just before that, though, nobody was going to the hospitals because it was a waste of time. There was nothing there.

Sometimes I'd go round the villages and see a baby or an adult who was desperately ill, and I'd say 'That baby needs to go into hospital. I'm going there tonight, and I'll take the baby with me.' But you had to be very careful, because they had to pay, and you had to make certain that they understood that although you'd take somebody in you weren't going to pay for the treatment. But almost invariably they'd refuse to come, and they'd say 'I'll speak to my husband', who wasn't going to be in until goodness knows when, or 'I'll wait till tomorrow', and you could see by the look on their faces that they weren't going to move that person.

The hospital staff seemed to have no compassion or understanding or sympathy at all. They were quite hard in their outlook. One of our babies was admitted with encephalitis, and when I went in he was lying on top of a formica table, and had been there for two hours. The nurse wasn't desperately busy with somebody else; she was just sitting there writing records. The mother was going to take the baby back to the village, because nothing was being done, and she'd been told 'If you want to take the baby back to the village, you *take* the baby back to the village.'

I said to the nurse 'Could you come a moment.' I had to be very careful because I had no *right* to say anything. I was just trying to smooth things over. Anyway, I eventually managed to get the baby taken off the formica table, and to be admitted, and to be given *some* kind of treatment. But they're not very sensitive or caring. Even my own lovely counterpart, Grace, had a very different outlook on things. Life is cheap there. Of necessity, it's cheap.

Most of the doctors and nurses *bought* their diplomas. They did their training, but the system was the same as in the schools. It didn't matter how hard pupils worked, or how clever they were, the teachers would fail them until they'd handed over a 'favour'. *Then* they'd be passed.

I found the Liberians very charming, *very* difficult to motivate, and absolutely corrupt. I think that's an African disease, but it's got to be worse in Liberia than anywhere else. That was very difficult to cope with.

Apart from the hospitals there were state clinics, but they had no drugs, nothing. They were run by practitioner assistants – PAs – who were the equivalent of an SRN, and most of them had run off with the funds a long time ago, so the clinics were mostly just a shell.

I once went to one of the clinics which happened to be in our training area. Our village health workers used to spend a week in a clinic so that they could see various patients under the guidance of the PA, and learn to diagnose certain conditions, and so on, and that's why I was there. The PA was away at the time. He was a scoundrel, and I didn't like him, and he was formally one of our *supervisors*, but we couldn't do anything about it, because he was quite a big nob in that area. Anyway, his assistant was there, who was a man with no qualifications, but a certain amount of experience, and while we were there a team from the World Health Organisation came round.

They said 'Do you do preventative medicine?' and this PA's assistant said 'Yes, yes. The mothers come in and we sit them down and tell them about the importance of breastfeeding,' and so on, and so on. I felt quite proud, because this was all being done under our guidance, and all the right answers were coming out.

Then WHO asked '*Why* do you tell them breastmilk is better?' And he said 'Well, if you're a kitten and drink cats' milk you become a cat, and if you're a calf and drink cows' milk you become a cow. So you mustn't give a baby cows' milk. If you did it would turn into a cow.'

If anybody needed blood they'd have to travel 60 miles to Monrovia to *buy* the empty bottle, and then they'd have to find somebody willing to provide the blood, and the donor would usually charge $20–25, which was a small fortune. They were very reluctant to give blood. Even a mother wouldn't give blood for her child. She'd go and ask all the cousins and uncles and everybody else. But a mother or father would *not* give blood. I couldn't get to the bottom of it.

TRYING TO CHANGE IT ALL

Originally we'd had the idea of taking on 16 villages, but Ada, who was good at working things out, because she was in the management field, said 'There's absolutely no way we're going to be able to do that with what we've got. It's got to be kept small.' So we took on six villages. We chose them with the help of the director of the hospital, because, obviously, we didn't know them.

We went out three times. The first visit was in order to introduce ourselves, and to explain what primary health care was all about, and to ask whether they'd be interested, and, if so, whether they'd form a committee to get things going. On the second visit we'd ask to meet the committee, and ask them to choose somebody to become a village health worker, and to choose a traditional birth attendant to come to us for training.

We gave them quite strong guidelines to follow in choosing these people, because they'd be inclined to pick on their best-educated villagers – their 'book person' – and, of course, it's the 'book person' who's most likely to run off with all the money, or to go off to Monrovia, or wherever, once he feels he's 'trained'. It was very difficult getting them to understand that these weren't the ideal people for the job, and we felt we couldn't interfere too much, because if anything went wrong we didn't want them turning round and saying 'Well, *you* chose him!'

We asked for two TBAs, and one of them had to be the eldest, even if she was 80–odd, because she'd be the head woman in midwifery, and couldn't be ignored. In fact, we held a workshop for all the TBAs who hadn't been chosen for the full training, and gave them a crash course, and supplied them with the kit we gave all our trained midwives, just so that they shouldn't feel left out. We didn't want any rivalry. I don't think there was any. Their kits contained soap, and a brush, and razors, and cord ties, and alcohol, and vitamin tablets, and a plastic mac. We tried to keep it as basic as possible.

VILLAGE HEALTH WORKERS

We'd select a village as a training centre, and have the VHWs (village health workers) there for three months. To start with we'd ferry them home every weekend, but soon discovered that was using too much of our petrol, so, later, we took them home just once a month.

We had a variety of Liberians to help with the teaching, like health inspectors, somebody from the vaccination team, midwives, PAs, and so on. So we had a course on teaching them how to teach, and they helped in drawing up the curriculum. I and Ada taught one or two subjects, but the rest was done by Liberians, and that went quite well.

At the outset I wanted them to concentrate on preventative medicine and environmental hygiene – getting the villagers to organise the digging of wells, which were desperately needed because contaminated water was one of the highest causes of mortality, advising on nutrition, that kind of thing. But it soon became obvious that the villagers weren't responding. They wanted their VHWs to offer treatment, and not just refer the sick to the nearest clinic, which might be 60 miles away. They wanted him to *do* something. Otherwise they'd go back to the black beggar.

So after we'd discovered what was going on I brought them back for a further workshop in the basics of using antibiotics – telling them of the dangers, and why they must follow a full course, and which antibiotic was best for what. They were going to the market and buying antibiotics anyhow, so that they *could* respond to the demand, although they'd never admit it. I'm sure the misuse of antibiotics must have been responsible for generating a lot of resistance.

The VHWs were very, very good. They were highly stimulated during the training, and after their lectures on wells they'd go back and speak to the people, and the whole community would get together, and they'd dig their wells, and they'd go round and clear the compound, and make sure their garbage dumps were in the right place. In one particular instance the chief called the villagers together, and suggested that no more graves should be dug within the compound, and that was good, because the community had got together and decided on that for itself.

One of the basic things the VHWs learned was how to treat diarrhoea with sugar and salt solution. They took that on board very well.

They held clinics, twice a day, or once a day, or twice a week – however they could fit it in with looking after their own fields and affairs, and they knew about first aid, and how to cope with somebody who'd fallen off a palm tree, and things like that.

We did have some trouble with one local clinic. It wasn't a government clinic. It was run by a Catholic mission, and the sister in charge was excellent, and did a magnificent job, but every single patient who came to her – and it didn't matter *what* was the matter – got an injection, even if it was only a vitamin injection. I spoke to her about this, and she said that if they didn't have an injection they'd feel they hadn't had their money's worth. So that was very difficult for any VHW working nearby, because it didn't matter how much good advice and treatment the villagers got from him, they'd still go off to the clinic to get their injection, which is what they thought they needed.

Later on we decided not to operate in villages close to this clinic, because it was soul-destroying for the VHWs. One of our best men worked right next door, and he was very much into prevention and education. I'd drawn up some brightly-coloured posters on nutrition, and things like that, and he used these, and they were a great asset to the VHWs when it came to teaching their people the right approach to enjoying better health, but it was all defeated when they were encouraged to think that all their problems could be much more easily solved by getting an injection.

One of the biggest problems, which we hadn't really conquered by the time we left, was the question of how VHWs were to be compensated for their work. Originally we said to the committees

'*You* choose how you want to recompense him – whether you want to work in his field, or give him some small money.' But it didn't work out.

In fact it was very difficult to get the villagers to work as a committee at all. It was a totally alien thing for them to do. They would sit down and listen to their elders or their chief, but to get them to make their own decisions was very difficult. Some villages did operate good committees, but others were an absolute dead loss, and we decided it was all to do with the chief. If they had a good chief, and a good community spirit, they'd get somewhere.

Anyway, when we did our supervision trips we found that this compensation lark wasn't working out. The VHWs' main complaint was that they weren't getting any recompense, and they said they weren't going to continue unless they did. So in the end, and just before we left, we established a revolving drug fund. We'd give each VHW an initial supply of about $200–worth, free, and they'd sell them at a price which would bring in enough money to let them restock from us, plus a small profit, which they could keep. That worked very well. We said 'Don't price the drugs too high, because if you do, people aren't going to come to you.' Most of them were quite responsible and intelligent about it, and, hopefully, that scheme will go on working. I don't know.

I've learnt from speaking to other people who've worked in primary health care in other third world countries that this business of compensation is one of the biggest problems, and it seems to me that we have to go in with *stronger* guidelines, and not be quite so modern-minded in sitting back and saying 'Well, *you* must decide. *You* are the people who are going to run this thing.' They really, in some ways, *want* to be told what to do. We went in a little bit stronger on our later sensitisation visits, and it seemed to work better.

I've had letters from our VHWs. They're all doing very well. They've got a grant from another charity. They've got another car, and six motorbikes. The revolving drug scheme seems to be working. I think we've left them with a going concern.

THE VILLAGE MIDWIVES

We gave the TBAs (traditional birth attendants) an eight-week course. They were a completely different kettle of fish. The VHWs *had* been to school. They were 'book people' and we could converse, whereas these women just spoke their own tribal dialect. That's where I was so fortunate in having Grace, because she'd been a TBA before training as a midwife, and had a marvellous rapport with our pupils, which I would never, ever, have achieved. They accepted me as the 'white woman', and it doesn't matter how long you live and work in their communities, you're still the 'white woman'. I couldn't have spoken to them, and even Grace had to have an interpreter in some of the villages, because she didn't speak *all* the dialects. Language apart, she understood their culture, and was able to get across ideas in ways I couldn't have attempted.

We didn't succeed too well in promoting antenatal care. The women felt they had absolutely no need to see anybody while they were pregnant unless they had problems.

Initially we charged them something like 2 ½p for a week's supply of vitamin and iron tablets, but they wouldn't come. So I said 'OK, *give* them the tablets.' But still they wouldn't come.

We asked the TBAs 'Why not?' and they said 'Well, the woman's not ill. What's the point?' They couldn't see the point of coming and being palpated for no apparent reason at all, and that was a big disappointment, because that's when you can catch most of the problems, but we hadn't got over that by the time I left.

We did manage to make them aware of the dangers of pro-longed deliveries, and to recognise positions when the woman did eventually present herself, and they did accept the virtue of dealing properly with the cord, and of encouraging breastfeeding, and so on.

I never really talked to them about female circumcision. You couldn't tell them to stop it. It was something too deeply ingrained in their culture. The most you could do was encourage the use of clean techniques.

GRADUATES

The TBAs and the VHWs went back to their villages with a
greatly enhanced status. They asked us whether they could wear
uniforms, and we said of course they could, but they'd have to pay
for them. So they went back to the villages and discussed it, and
the villages got together and raised the money. They looked quite
smart. The VHWs had blue trousers and a blue tunic, and the
TBAs had a blue native gown and a headdress. UNICEF provided
us with a kit which they could all carry with them, and that was
a source of great pride.

At one of our graduation ceremonies we had the VHWs put on
a play, and it was about a young couple having problems with their
baby, who was dying, and they went to the medicine man. We had
a marvellous VHW who took this role, and he really looked very
good, and was throwing the stones, and doing all the abracadabra
stuff – telling this couple what they should do. And then a woman
in the audience came up, and she wanted *her* fortune told, and then
another man came up, and then another. And that was nearly the
end of my play. It was being taken over.

But they were very proud, with their uniforms and boxes
and diplomas.

LIVING IT UP

The British embassy took a great interest in us when we arrived
because we were the first VSOs in the country, and they provided
our first accommodation, which was a most magnificent house,
meant for a senior expatriate. I was bitterly disappointed, because
that wasn't what I'd gone out there for at all. We were stuck in
the middle of nowhere every weekend in this beautiful house, but
with no transport, and I felt as if I was in an open prison. It was
awful. I hated it, and became very despondent.

Then, after a year, I managed to find my own little mud hut
in the village, and I really loved it. I had some very nice Peace
Corps neighbours, as well as some helpful Liberians. There was

actually some *life* in the place. I could actually *see* people. That was my happiest time.

I say 'little mud hut', but it wasn't just a round thing with a hole in the roof to let the smoke out. It was a little up on the ordinary village hut. I had a large sitting room, fairly sparsely furnished, and a bedroom and kitchen and spare room, and a loo and shower at the back. The Peace Corps had lived there, and they'd fixed up the shower with a drum on the roof, so the water got quite warm from the sun. That was great.

The loo was awful. It was shaped like an ordinary lav, and had a proper lav seat, but it was just perched over a hole in the ground, and swarming with cockroaches. I was quite amazed, because I thought Americans were very, very finicky – how they could have used it was beyond me. But a lovely Peace Corps neighbour built me an S-shaped loo, which was beautiful.

There was the club, where expatriates used to go. Some used to go every week. We had barbecues there. So there was a certain amount of mixing.

I had quite enough money. VSOs are usually paid the local going rate for the job, and up until about four years before we arrived Liberian medical workers had been getting excellent pay – much better than here. Mind you, *that* doesn't take a lot of beating. Then the economic situation got worse and worse, and their pay got cut and cut. At one point they hadn't been paid at all for three months. So our salaries had to be negotiated with Plan, rather than simply being based on Liberian rates, and we were allowed $350 a month, which was, as it happens, the equivalent of what I was earning here.

I lived rent-free. I wasn't paying *any* bills. I was really living quite well, and kept myself well supplied with gin and cigarettes. In fact I was able to save an enormous sum of money. VSO would be horrified if they *knew* that.

I was visited by my daughter and her husband, and my mother.

I didn't take a break in the two years, which was probably a mistake, and I did end up counting the days. I think everybody does that. You may be enjoying it immensely, but you still start counting the days to coming back.

The humidity got me down eventually – that and the mosquitoes. And I missed the theatre. I go to the theatre a lot.

I was quite surprised to find, after getting back, that I *didn't* have itchy feet. I thought I'd be longing to go back there again. But I'm really very, very happy to be back.

My daughter said 'Now you've done it at *your* age, I know *I* can go out and do it.'

British nurses are highly valued in North America. An RGN is reckoned to be at least as good as a native 'graduate' nurse, and since they're getting short of nurses over there too (for reasons which will emerge below) great efforts are made to tempt our own Nightingales to have a go in the New World, where they can earn up to three times more money.

The comments which follow were garnered at a 'nursing jobs fair' staged in London in the summer of 1987. Representatives from some 20 American hospitals and medical agencies had gathered at the Novotel Hotel in Hammersmith, hoping to recruit several hundred would-be émigrés, before moving on to Eire where the pickings were expected to be even richer. An earlier campaign mounted by Australians from Victoria had procured 500 British nurses for the state, from among 3,500 who'd responded to advertisements.

The Hammersmith event generated a good deal of publicity in the papers and on telly, prompting Mrs Edwina Currie, a junior health minister in the Thatcher administration, to claim that nurses swallowing the American bait might become sadly disillusioned with the reality. Salaries might be high, she said, but they'd find accommodation a lot more expensive, they'd have no NHS to succour them when ill, and they'd have to pay to put their children through college. 'It isn't necessarily a better world over there.' The ladies from the other side I spoke to seemed to think she was talking through her pretty little hat.

Any nurses offered a post have to pass a 'foreign nurse exam', taken in the UK, and are then issued a temporary permit for work in the USA. Some time after arrival they have to pass a further exam in order to be registered within the employing state. It seems that no British RGN need fear such hurdles.

Kathleen Clarke, not a nurse herself, is manager of nurse recruitment for Harper Hospital in Detroit. This 917 bed teaching institution is one of a group of seven hospitals forming the Detroit Medical Center – the largest such complex in Michigan.

We've spoken to a number of English nurses who are interested in coming to the States, and many of them have expressed some discontent with their lot, if you will. But the interesting thing is that I've also spoken to a number of *parents*, enquiring on behalf of their daughters, and *they've* said they don't think English nurses are held in proper respect, and aren't treated as professonals, and are underpaid and overworked.

I've just had one young lady in who gave me an example of this. She was the only registered nurse working on a 32–bed orthopaedic ward, and she had one SEN to help. She asked me how many patients a nurse would have under her care in the US. When I said it would depend on how ill the patients were, but that as a general rule it would be about six, she was astounded. In critical care it's one-to-one, and we would close beds if we don't have that ratio.

Some have been worried that they might find living in the States terribly expensive, and I've read what your minister had to say about that, but it just isn't true. We've sat down and compared notes, and when we've added it all up we've found it's cheaper to live in Michigan than London by a *long* way. I've said 'If you come to Michigan you really have to have a car.' And they say 'How could we *ever* afford a car?' Then I explain that it's really very easy. You can get a car for a little more than £100 a month, but you're making at least £1,250 a month.

We haven't signed anybody on. We haven't had any formal interviews. They just need to know something about us. They'll get their questions answered, and they'll take our literature, and then they'll come back, or we'll correspond. I don't want to get anyone over there on false pretences. I don't want to raise their expectations and have them dashed.

WHY BOTHER?

British nurses are considered to be *very* well trained, which is why we'd like to have them. We're not desperate yet. We'd be happy if we got ten here, and we expect to find perhaps 20 when we go to Dublin next week. So we're not desperate, but we can see what's coming.

Our nursing school enrolment is down 20 per cent. Young people aren't going into nursing in the same numbers as they were. Part of that is the population trend, and part is the fact that there are so many other professions women now feel free to enter. And then, when you've been in nursing for a couple of years, there are so many opportunities open to you, away from the ward. There's a position called clinical nurse specialist you can study for. That requires a master's degree. We have nurses in research who are PhDs.

You can become a nurse recruiter. You can work for a pharmaceutical firm. You can teach at university or community-college level. Utilisation review is another area. Insurance companies will hire nurses to go out and look at the way hospitals administer their insurance programmes. They will look at the sort of surgery going on, and whether policies and procedures are producing good results.

Some go into home health care. A few get attached to weight-loss clinics, and other popular health-for-sale ventures, which seem to think they'll gain prestige by having a qualified nurse on the staff. That's frowned upon by nurses who like to consider themselves to be professionals.

But there are just so many areas nurses can go into.

Some leave the field altogether, perhaps to raise a family, or perhaps because of what we call 'burn out'. That mostly happens among nurses working in critical care areas, where you may be making life-and-death decisions ten times a day, and it all becomes too much.

We do give women who've left to raise a family the option of coming back to work for one day a week, or a couple of hours a day, if they wish. I understand you don't have that option here.

WORK FOR THE LISTENING BOSS

Some of the girls I've seen have complained that nobody listens to their problems and suggestions, and I've told them about *our* set-up.

We have staff nurse councils. We have a recruitment committee, and we have a retention committee, so that the staff nurses are getting together, not so much to air grievances, but to work out how they can make the job better. 'We need to move *this* bit of equipment, or we need to knock out *that* wall, and then we can do a better job.' They define the problem and suggest the solution, and then they're supported by the administration who say 'Yes, you're right. We'll *do* that for you.'

I think that's something nurses in the UK lack. They're not feeling *cared* for. They're not feeling *listened* to.

Theresa Broderick is a nurse manager, the equivalent of a sister, and runs a 40–bed unit. Like every nurse I've spoken to, she loves her job. She gave much the same reasons as her countrywoman, Kathleen Clarke, for the nursing shortage in the USA, but had some interesting extra comments to make concerning Mrs Currie's claim that nurses going to the USA might find themselves in a financial mess.

A person needs to be adventurous to come over. But we're not trying to recruit people and just drop them into our society 'cold'. We really have thought about it, and how we can have the English come over and feel very comfortable. The hospitals cover an employee's health insurance, and that should not be a concern.

The cost of living depends on where you live. I find London very expensive, like New York City, but I live in South Jersey, and our cost of living is not high at all. When nurses come over they have the choice of where to live. If they want to live in the city centre it *will* cost them money, but the suburbs are cheaper. They don't *have* to live in the hospital, or even close by, if they don't want to.

We've had an overwhelming response – a lot of interest and a lot of questions. Quite a few married women with children are interested in coming over on a temporary basis, whereas we were thinking our population would be more along the single line. And we've had a lot of enquiries from SENs, but unfortunately our immigration laws don't allow us to recruit them at this point. They don't have enough education to be a registered nurse in our country.

I love nursing, and one of the benefits I very much appreciate is that if you want to get any further education the hospital pays your tuition. We have to pay for our college training. It's not like your country, where it's free. I paid for my undergraduate degree, and then went to work in hospitals that paid 100 per cent tuition. So I got my master's degree without paying a penny, which is very nice, because it *is* expensive if you have to pay for it yourself. Hospitals realise this, and they want their nurses to get as much more education as they wish, so they say 'OK, we'll pay for it.' I love that. It's great.

It's very easy to advance your career in the States. As a matter of fact, I'm trying to talk my brother into becoming a nurse. He's at college right now. He was going to be a teacher, but he's a bit concerned because our teachers don't get paid that much money. Nurses' salaries are well above our teachers' salaries. He's realised that as a nurse he could teach as well. So he's quite interested.

Mary O'Kane trained at the Westminster Hospital and became a theatre sister. She went to the USA for a 'working holiday' 12 years ago, and has been there ever since. She works in, and was recruiting for, a county hospital which caters for the indigent sick who don't have health insurance, and 'are used for teaching'.

I like travelling. I wanted to see the States properly and decided that the only way I could afford that was by working there. I was planning to come back after a year and then go somewhere else. But at the end of the year I was having a really good time, so I thought I'd stay for another six months, and then another six months, and I'm still there.

I particularly like the physician/nurse relationship. There's a lot of camaraderie, and you're very much part of the team. You're involved in a lot of the planning that goes on during surgery and all that, and that's what I like.

I'm regarded as a professional in my own right. I'm not expected to be a handmaiden. Some of the doctors I've worked with here in the UK were awfully nice, but some just treated me as their maid. They didn't seem to think I was worth acknowledging as a person. I'm not saying there aren't any American doctors like that. I've come across some physicians with the God complex in the private sector, where I first worked, and which I didn't enjoy at *all*.

The other thing I like is the fact that I've plenty of chance for promotion, and to better myself. They pay for you to study. I go out to study at college, part-time, at night, and they pay so much of my tuition. They do push a lot over there for people to get their bachelor's degree in nursing, but I feel I *am* a nurse already, and I'm aiming to do a degree in management. Then I could go into an administrative position in nursing, but there are also lots of companies that will take health-care people on as consultants or whatever, and that's the sort of job I have in mind. I'd like that.

I wouldn't say nurses are given more responsibility in the States. I can remember that when I first went there I couldn't *believe* that I wasn't allowed to give somebody a paracetamol tablet without calling the doctor. On the other hand we start up intravenous infusions, which doesn't happen here, and we do arterial jabs. It evens out.

Nurses there are fighting for more autonomy. If they don't get it, they'll leave.

I come back to Britain all the time to visit. I don't think I'll ever come back here to live. Not unless British nurses somehow become a much superior kind of being.

Chapter 9

THE QUEEN - GOD BLESS HER

A good many women, and a few men, find happiness in serving their Queen and country as nurses within one of the armed forces of the Crown.

It all started with Florence Nightingale, of course (didn't everything?), for after her Scutari adventure the idea of having nurses specially devoted to the care of sick and wounded soldiers stuck. The army and the navy began to employ their own small nursing corps, and in 1902 Queen Alexandra bestowed her royal patronage upon the breed, thereafter named Queen Alexandra's Imperial Military Nursing Service and Queen Alexandra's Royal Naval Nursing Service.

For historical reasons beyond the scope of this book, but not unrelated to Ghandi, India, and all that, the 'Imperial' bit was dropped from the military nurses' title in 1949, and the two services are now popularly known as the QAs and the QUARNS. The RAF missed out on Alexandra, and their nurses come under the mantle of Princess Mary. They are members of PMRAFNS – the PMs.

Life as a nurse in any of the three services seems to be much the same, and within the past few years they've all come under a central directorate at the Ministry of Defence which controls broad policies, but below that level they clearly cherish their separate identities and traditions. Thus a recruiting brochure for the naval lot claims that 'compared to outfits in any of the other Services' the uniform of a female trainee is 'one of the most attractive'. (There *are* only two other services!)

The QAs present a slightly more macho image than the QUARNS, which is understandable, since military nurses are rather more likely to get close to fighting and turmoil on the ground. Naval nurses don't go to sea, except, perhaps, in a hospital ship – a rare and temporary being. (The Royal Yacht, which is so designed, was converted for use as a hospital during the Falklands affair.) Any nursing duties required afloat are undertaken by medical assistants (the old sick-berth attendants), who are not part of the QUARNS, although nursing officers play an important part in their training.

During her initial training every QA goes for early morning jogs, works in the gym, and experiences the delights of an assault course. She must be able to run half-a-mile in six minutes, and a mile and a half in $13^3/_4$ minutes – not a demand to strain the capacity of any but the slowest and heaviest of mortals. QUARNS and PMs are simply promised 'a fair amount of saluting and marching and plenty of work in the gymnasium'.

Owing to the dissolution of the Empire, overseas postings are neither so varied nor so numerous as they used to be, and a QUARN could spend her entire career in the UK, although there is one small naval hospital in Gibraltar (largely a maternity unit), and occasionally an officer with a specialist qualification will be loaned to another service for a job abroad. A QA will certainly spend some time in Germany, and could go to Northern Ireland, Cyprus, Hong Kong, the Falklands, and even Nepal.

All three services accept men and women with the necessary academic qualifications to join as 'rankers' for RGN training. Qualified SENs can also join the ranks. SEN training is no longer provided, thanks to the dead hand of Project 2000. Officers are RGNs who have achieved direct entry by passing a selection board, or rankers who have qualified as RGNs within the service and then been chosen for promotion – by no means an automatic process.

Miss E.M. Northway is Matron-in-Chief of the QUARNS. She joined the service in 1956, feeling the need to 'spread my wings' and because 'the sea was in my blood'.

I think I'd always wanted to be a nurse, but I also seemed to want to have something to do with one of the services, and the Navy seemed to be the one that I wanted to have something to do with. My grandfather was a master seaman, and two of my uncles were in the Navy. Added to that, during the war, and when I was very young, the Navy took over a big hospital in Newton Abbot, in Devon, where I was born, and I used to see these nursing sisters crossing the road, and I rather thought I'd like the uniform.

I trained in Torquay, because my mother wouldn't let her only daughter go further afield. I then did my midwifery and, having got my qualifications, applied for the Navy because I thought I'd have some involvement with the sea. But, of course, we don't.

I joined the naval hospital in Plymouth. We didn't train nurses in those days. The service was composed of nursing officers and sick-berth attendants, and we still had some VADs (Voluntary Aid Detachments, supplied by the Red Cross – mostly 'ladies' wanting to perform 'good works'), who did the mundane duties, if you like. I spent a year in Plymouth, and then went to a medical centre to look after WRENS. That was a kind of general practice, with a small in-patient facility to look after minor illnesses and injuries. And after that to the naval hospital in Hong Kong, which was a very busy and enjoyable two years.

In those days we were required to be exceedingly adaptable, and leap from doing surgical nursing to medical nursing to whatever. I may be quite wrong to say this, at least in the eyes of some of my senior colleagues in the NHS, but I believe those days were far better than they are now, because nurses could turn their hands to anything. It's fine that people are specialising, but I think that if they get too deeply involved in a narrow field, difficulties occur. In Hong Kong we dealt with all kinds of nursing problems, ranging from tropical diseases to injuries incurred by sailors falling down ladders, and we also looked after families – children and wives.

After Hong Kong I did a whole variety of jobs, here and abroad, including running a ward at Haslar in Gosport for three years. Then to Malta to look after a community project we ran for service wives. Then back here to another medical centre, then back to hospital, including a spell in an accident and emergency unit at Haslar. And then I began to be taken out of direct nursing.

I went off to a drafting establishment and was responsible for the movement of non-commissioned medical personnel, which included nurses and the male medical assistants, drafting them to ships and the Royal Marines. That was a very interesting job, and I didn't really think I could do it, but in fact I managed.

Then back to Haslar as deputy matron for a couple of years, and then matron, but that didn't last long, because I got promoted and went into pure administration.

As Matron-in-Chief now I'm responsible to the Medical Director General (MDG) for the standards of nursing care provided for patients in naval hospitals, and for the welfare and training of personnel within the QUARNS. To achieve that I have to liaise with the civilian statutory bodies, and follow their rules and regulations. That kind of career doesn't happen to a lot of people now, unfortunately, because we've become so small.

I have nursing officers now doing what we call staff jobs – working with medical officers in administrative roles. Some people get very cross and upset about that, but I believe that if we want to promote our profession, then we have to demonstrate that we're capable of appreciating and influencing the wider aspects of medical care, and are not just concerned with practical nursing. Having said that, in no way must we let our standards on the nursing side drop. But we have to make absolutely sure that the profession is recognised *as* a profession.

Nursing has come a very long way since I did my training. When I think of the slave labour! We didn't really grumble about it, because we didn't know anything else. But medical technology is becoming more sophisticated, so the people looking after the patients have to be more knowledgeable. Very often, in the old days, we didn't understand how to apply what we'd learnt in the schools to the practical situation. You were taught one way in the school of nursing, and then you were let loose on a ward and, because of the sheer busy-ness and the activity and all the rest of it, you couldn't actually do things in the way you'd been taught you should do them. I think those days are going away.

OTHER RANKS

In 1962 we were given approval to do our own nurse training. We did have a very small school of nursing of our own in Portsmouth, but in 1982, because of the changes in nursing taking place, we thought it would be politic to merge with the local NHS school, which is now called the Portsmouth and Royal Naval School of Nursing, and that's benefitted both of us. Our students get practical experience in the RN hospital for much of their time, but go to civilian hospitals for training we can't provide, like geriatrics. We get an inspection from the English National Board every five years to make sure our training is up to the mark.

We can't train too many because we're restricted with our nurse manpower these days, but at the moment we take 20 a year, and that'll be up to 25 next year. They may do one or two years as a staff nurse after they've qualified, and within that time they may have the opportunity to gain another qualification, such as an operating theatre diploma, or a certificate in intensive care. Unfortunately the number we can now send on courses is very limited, because of cuts.

We used to train enrolled nurses, but when we merged with the Portsmouth NHS school that ended. They'd stopped their EN course because of Project 2000 coming in. SENs actually form the backbone of our nursing support, and now we're very short of them, and they're very disturbed about their future. I think they've been demoralised.

I think a great mistake was made in phasing out enrolled nurses. Since we stopped training them we've been recruiting direct-entry enrolled nurses, but we haven't achieved our target. The services have a great need for a second-level nurse. I think the mistake was the rather instantaneous decision that enrolled nurse training should go. It's all happened too quickly.

The UKCC has said that SENs' futures must be looked after, and that conversion courses must be provided, but in my experience they *cannot* get conversion courses.

We've been training *one* enrolled nurse every other year to RGN standard, and from next year we hope to train three a year, which is actually quite good, considering we're a very small service. If we can do that every year, that will boost the morale of our existing SENs and, hopefully, let them see some hope for the future. I do know there's a lot of unhappiness among enrolled nurses because they simply don't know where they are. It's all very well saying conversion courses will be available. But they're *not*. Not in the numbers required by the girls wanting to do it.

Whilst I agree that it's marvellous to envisage a practitioner nurse – a one-level nurse, a specialist nurse – this idea of the 'helper' to look after the chores worries me, because at some stage that helper is going to want some recognition. It's back to the 1950s, when we had state enrolled assistant nurses, who got that title because they had x number of years of experience in hospitals. I can't remember the year when the course became formalised, and they took exams, but the whole thing came about because the assistant nurses wanted a badge and a certificate and recognition – something to say that *she* was a qualified nurse. I think that's going to happen with the 'helper', eventually. I think the whole thing will go full circle.

The medical assistants are the responsibility of the head of the medical services branch, but they *are* taught in our school of nursing, and our tutors do get involved in their curriculum, and their expertise has enhanced the MAs' training. MAs do a year's course which includes working in medical and surgical wards, and an accident and emergency department, and the operating theatre. They also do a week with a local ambulance service. So they acquire medical and surgical and first-aid skills, combined with naval training. It's a very comprehensive course. They have to be trained to a level at which they can function for five days afloat without a medical officer, because not all ships have an MO, although there's always radio contact. They end up with a City & Guilds certificate, but it's a non-statutory training, not recognised by the Central Council. Some do manage to use their qualifications when they leave by going on oil rigs and such places, or maybe joining an ambulance service.

We've just introduced a female medical assistant. They won't go to sea, and I'm seeing them as our second-level nurses – our 'helpers' – in the long term.

We don't *want* to replace the enrolled nurse, but it's being forced upon us. We do *need* a person who's sufficiently trained in first aid and general ward and patient-care skills to be able to work under minimal supervision, because we have these medical centres to manage.

Our requirement is different to that of the NHS. Not so much in the hospitals, perhaps, but we have to have people trained to function comprehensively in peace *and* war. That's why we're here. We don't *want* war. None of us does. But it's only right that there should be an efficient nursing service to look after soldiers, sailors and airmen, so that they can be dealt with quickly when they're injured, or whatever, and be returned quickly to duty.

Our main area of concern now is the enrolled nurse shortage. I think it's sad.

OFFICERS

We have 103 nursing officers at the moment, and that includes me. There are about 365 nurses, including those in training. We're the smallest service.

I hold interview boards on average every other month for civilian applicants for commissions. They must have two years' post-registration experience, and preferably another qualification, but that's not essential. They have to pass a fairly stiff inquisition. We use the Admiralty Interview Board in Gosport. I'm the president, and then there'll be a matron, a senior doctor representing the MDG, and a senior naval officer.

Whenever we interview people, whether they want to come in as an officer or a rating, we always ask 'Why do you want to join the Navy?' and invariably they'll say 'We like the idea of a disciplined organisation, because we'll *know* where we are.'

We look for all sorts of things, and not just their qualifications. We're looking for leadership qualities, the right personality traits, intelligence, and commitment. By that I mean, what have they done to find out about the service they're asking to join? I want to make sure their interest isn't just a passing fancy. I've already looked at their references, so the interview is the decider. We can only take 12 a year, so I can be very selective about who we see, and the board is selective too, which means we really take the best.

We see four candidates at each two-monthly session, and that includes our own NCOs applying for promotion. Sometimes we accept them all, and sometimes they're *all* a disaster, but on average we'll accept about 70 per cent. We treat civilian applicants and our own people in exactly the same way. We turn down quite a few of our own, because a lot of them are very good staff nurses, but wouldn't make good nursing officers. So the whole thing's very fair.

Afterwards I see any we've rejected, privately, and say 'I'm very sorry you've failed. It's probably due to this, that and the other thing. If you like to go away and broaden your experience and apply again I'll be pleased to interview you.' Because lack of experience is usually one of the reasons for failure on the civilian side.

I just recently had one of our own male staff nurses up for a second go. He was very keen to become an officer, but didn't perform terribly well at his first board. We all felt his overwhelming aim was to become an officer – full stop. When I talked to him afterwards he denied that, but after talking to him quite a bit, it became clear that that *was* his intention. He *wanted* to be an *officer*. I pointed out that, at the end of the day, being an officer on the nursing side was fine, but he mustn't just think of it in that context. He went away, and after a year we saw him again, and his reports were very good, and he's been accepted.

He's not been promoted yet, because once someone's been passed by the board we have to go through another selection procedure up here, and appointments depend on the number of places available in the financial year, and so on. We've 12 male nursing officers at the moment.

THE CAREER

Officers come in on an initial five-year short-service commission. At any time after three years they can apply to have that extended to eight, which is where the short-term commission ends.

Some time between their fifth and sixth year they can apply for a pensionable medium-career commission, which is a total of 16 years' service. Whether that's granted depends on the number of places available (which is particularly pertinent these days), and on their suitability. They have to come up here and be interviewed by me and the MDG's representative at a board which meets once a year. We test their knowledge of the service, and so forth, and marry that up with their confidential annual reports.

Beyond that there's the chance of a full career commission, which means they can carry on until they reach the retiring age of the rank they're holding. They start in the rank of nursing officer, and then to senior nursing officer, superintending nursing officer, chief nursing officer (the matrons), and principal nursing officer, for the broader administrative jobs. Unfortunately, because of the narrow promotion pinnacle, we've now got quite a lot of superintending nursing officers who know they won't get any further. The retiring age for them and for matrons is 53. A PNO goes at 55.

There are five matrons – two at Haslar, one at Plymouth, one in Gibraltar, and one up here as my deputy. Soon we'll have a sixth as an in-service training officer, looking after the post-basic training element for the whole service.

So things have changed quite a lot since I joined. Then we had three naval hospitals in the UK and four overseas. Now competition for the senior posts is *very* fierce. With such a small service we have to be, and can afford to be, highly selective.

Before January 1984 each arm of the services had its own medical directorate, headed by a director-general who was a vice-admiral, or its equivalent, and a matron-in-chief who was a commodore. Now we have a combined Defence Medical Services Directorate, with *one* head of medical services and *one* director of nursing. We are still, in effect, separate services at command level, but HQ determines general policies. That meant a step-down in rank for some of the nursing and medical chiefs, but the two senior posts, retaining the old top ranks, go round the three services in rotation. You still have to be the best person for the job. The two things have to marry up.

THE LIFE

There's a lot of motivation among the nursing staff. They're very professional, and they're suitably trained on the service side to enable them to fit in with the RN administration. That really is where the difference between NHS and services nursing ends, because nursing, wherever you go, is the same, and we do look after a percentage of civilian patients.

They like nursing in the services because we do have a structured system. Everybody knows who their boss is, and there's a regulated promotion system for both officers and NCOs.

They practise nursing of all descriptions. Mainly general medicine and surgery and orthopaedics, but we also have intensive care units – coronary care – and accidents and emergencies. Along the way one gets involved in service functions and service discipline, which makes the whole thing very interesting. You're really having two careers.

You know what your pathway is. You get told at regular intervals whether you're doing well, or not doing well, and whether you're going to make it. I think that's very fair. I think people *should* know that. Everybody knows where they can go if they have a problem. In the navy we have the divisional system. An officer is responsible for a body of ratings – usually those he or she is working with. So a ward nursing officer is responsible for running that ward, and is also responsible for her ratings staff on that ward. She is responsible for their welfare, and for keeping them up to date with current conditions of service or regulations, and for fighting on their behalf. If they get themselves into trouble she is their 'friend', if you like. And if she feels there's a problem to do, say, with a particular condition of service, she can make that known to the executive commander in the hospital, who would forward it to MoD for solution.

At HQ there's a Directorate of Naval Service Conditions. They look after everybody's welfare, and we all know how to approach them. There's a well-defined route for channelling suggestions and complaints. So on the personnel side there aren't the bureaucratic barriers to communication that you have, perhaps, within the NHS. In fact, I think we go to extreme lengths to ensure that everybody's fairly treated. Everybody has a chance, and if they don't take it, that's their fault.

Although we're becoming more and more restricted, because of defence cuts, we still have quite a lot to offer, and most of our nurses enjoy what they're doing. All right – they may get frustrated because we say to them 'You'll have to manage with what you've *got*' (and I think they manage extremely well), but there are bonuses to being in the service.

It used to be that they got more pay, and more opportunity for travel. I don't think there's a tremendous difference in the pay now between the armed nursing services and the NHS, but it's the *environment*, and the sticking to tradition – providing tradition doesn't hamper progress – and it doesn't seem to have done that with us.

We don't have many drop-outs.

I've enjoyed my career. I don't know whether I'm enjoying it quite so much now. There's a lot of frustration in a position like this, and sometimes it's rather difficult to see light at the end of the tunnel. But I'm actually very proud of my set-up. My nurses do an extremely good job, and they're highly motivated, and on the whole, I think, very happy. Because they know where they are.

You'd probably find three or four saying 'No – we *don't* know where we are.' Some people *never* know where they are.

Sue Potter was matron/administrator of Bourn Hall Clinic near Cambridge when I spoke to her. This is where the late Mr Patrick Steptoe and Dr Robert Edwards established an internationally-celebrated centre for the generation of 'test-tube babies'. She is now matron of a newly-established children's hospice, also near Cambridge, where physically and mentally disabled young people can be nursed for a time while their families take a break, and which aims to provide support for parents faced with the emotionally and physically demanding task of caring for heavily dependent children.

She spent the better part of the first half of her professional career with the QAs, and is proof of the fact that service life can provide a pretty good foundation for all kinds of quite different efforts.

I wanted to nurse sick children from a very young age, and I wrote to Great Ormond Street when I was only 12 to see if I could train there. The only stumbling block was that they wanted five O levels, and I could *not* pass maths. It was the geometry that always stumped me, and I failed three times. Finally they said they'd take me if I could pass the Royal Society of Arts arithmetic exam, and that was no trouble, so I finally started there a couple of weeks after my 18th birthday. That was on 30 December 1963. I always remember that date very clearly.

When I got there I found we were the first set to undertake the four-year combined training course, which none of us knew about before we arrived. But in those days you were just *told* what you were going to do. We had no choice. We had to do three years' children's nursing, and then they'd send us somewhere else for a fourth year of general training.

I thought 'Crikey!' Three years seemed a long time, and four-and-a-half years seemed endless, but I did realise it was the way to do it. So I had three years at GOS and then a year at the London. It was a jolly hard training, and wasn't at all how I'd imagined it to be. It was very much harder in all ways, both physically and emotionally.

One time at GOS I'll never forget was the fortnight we had to spend in the milk kitchen. We had a 15-minute coffee break. We had to leave the kitchen, take off our clothing, get over to the nurses' home, and be back in 15 minutes dressed up again. We never *had* a cup of coffee. It was too hot. You couldn't drink it. And in that milk kitchen we actually had to *dry* the rubber bands.

I remember being terrified on night duty when the staff nurse was taking her meal break, and there'd just be two of us students left in a ward of 20 beds with some very ill children. There was always somebody you could call, but it was still frightening. We used to sit making cotton-wool balls on night duty. You get them out of a packet now.

ARMY LIFE

I'd enjoyed my student days in many ways, but we were only earning £13 a month, and toward the end I was attracted by adverts for the QAs in the nursing press, because of the salary and the travelling. And I wanted to put off deciding what to do for a time.

I joined the QAs on a two-year commission and was posted to Aldershot. But when I got there I found that some people on a two-year engagement spent their entire time there, and I thought I might as well have gone to the Aldershot General. So I extended my commitment, and within three months I was in Germany, and three months after that I was in Singapore. Things really took off.

I worked with children from the start, and was finally in charge of a 70–bed ward in Singapore. We had a lot of local children – Malays and Indians as well as British – and that was very interesting. It was also my first experience of a general ward where there were all kinds of cases, medical and surgical, mixed together.

It was there I first realised that hospital isn't necessarily the best place for some children who need care but who aren't really ill. They'd be better off without the hustle and bustle and the strict routine which has to be enforced for the good of all the patients.

When I came back from Singapore I was about 25, and realised it was time to make up my mind about how I was going to spend my life. While I was on leave I went to look for a job at Addenbrooke's Hospital in Cambridge, because my parents live in Essex. But there was something about the place I didn't like. There was an atmosphere I didn't like. It was impersonal, and it was sloppy. The nurses all wore different shoes, for instance, and they *looked* sloppy. It's so big. You walked around and nobody took any notice. You could have had green hair for all they cared. And that great chimney! You wonder what they burn in their incinerator.

I thought 'Well, *this* won't do. I've got to make my mind up.' So I applied for a regular commission. You can serve for up to eight years as a short-service officer, and after that you either have to become a regular officer or go. At the end of my fifth year I applied for a 16–year commission, which is the earliest you *can* leave without affecting your pension. I'd never imagined I'd stay in the QAs as long as I did, but I didn't leave until 1984. I had two years in Hong Kong, two in Singapore, and three postings in Germany, totalling six or seven years, so the greater part of my time was spent overseas.

Because we had student nurses in these places we were not only dealing with sick children and their families, but also young boys or girls who were away from home for the first time. So it was a very caring role. You tried to establish a rapport with everybody working on your ward, whether it was the cleaner, who might be a local German lady, or a homesick student, or a newly-qualified sister who also needed help. It was very enjoyable to work in a team like that.

Some people imagine that a military hospital must be a stiff and formal place with lots of discipline. I don't think the discipline's very different from that in any other hospital. You'd have the commanding officer's inspection once a week, and even if he did have a sharp eye for cleanliness and hygiene, that would be for the patients' sake, and no more than you'd expect from any good ward sister.

The patients are just the same. A good proportion of them are young, so they'll be extra cheeky, and will think they can get away with it, just because they're in hospital.

Free visiting for the parents of sick children was introduced very soon after that idea was first suggested, and the nurses in children's wards wear tabards, so that they don't appear strange and fearsome. We tried to keep up.

If it wasn't for the uniforms around, I don't think you'd know you were in a military hospital. But you're all part of a great big team. Whether you met a cook or a quartermaster or a cleaner, you'd say 'Hello' or 'Good morning' or whatever. That's what I liked. Not like Addenbrooke's.

It was a very full life. When I was in Singapore we used to hire a car and go up to Malaya for weekends, and see the turtles on the beaches, and the white sand, too hot to walk on, and all so deserted in those days.

I enjoyed my time in the QAs very much, but I left at the end of my 16 years, in the rank of major, because I didn't want to travel around, packing my trunks, until I was 55 or 60. I wanted to settle, and have my own home, and a garden with roses, and a dog.

You can't have a dog when you're in the QAs.

AMBITION THWARTED

Early on I'd had this idea that hospital is the wrong place for a lot of children who need basic care, but who aren't ill – brain-damaged children, and so on. Perhaps we saw a lot of them in military hospitals abroad, because the families hadn't got the back-up of grannies and aunties and the rest, so these children came to us when the parents couldn't cope. But I felt they didn't want all this hustle and bustle of a hospital ward, and should have a special kind of refuge of their own.

While I was in Hong Kong, near the end of my service, I read about Helen House, in Oxford, which opened in the early '80s as the first children's hospice, and I went there to visit on my next leave to England, and found it was just the kind of place I'd had in mind for years.

I wanted to establish another one like it, and a year before leaving the QAs I wrote to a lot of local health authorities in the Essex area, which is where I wanted to settle, near my parents, suggesting the idea. I didn't get very far, because although I went to see all the right officials in places like Hertford and Harlow and Cambridge, nobody wanted actually to fund such a scheme.

All right – they'd got children they'd be happy to send to a place like that tomorrow, and yes, it *was* needed – but no money.

Oh dear!

So then I thought I'd write to various charities, and they all wrote back saying 'Why don't you go and work in a children's home?' and so on and so forth. Much sympathy, but 'Sorry we can't help financially.'

Oh dear!

TEST-TUBE BABIES

At this stage I left the QAs and had a couple of months doing agency work before seeing the Bourn Hall matron's job advertised. That appealed to me, because it's a small unit where you know all the patients and all the staff – not like Addenbrooke's. I came here as matron in 1984, and the following year the administrator left, so I took over both positions as matron/manager.

It's been a very good experience for me. I've learnt how to run the budgeting side. Also we've been involved with the health authority, so now I know all the legal side of running an independent medical concern as well.

Some 40–50 per cent of our patients come from overseas and, having met all the different nationalities while in the QAs, it's nice to meet them here again as well. We do get a lot from the Middle East. Often the woman's marriage depends on her producing a baby, and preferably a son. If she doesn't, then the husband finds another wife. They're not ill, but they're under a lot of emotional strain. Very often it's their last resort – coming here to get pregnant. And they're paying for their treatment, so in some ways they expect more of you. They'll say the food isn't worth the money they're paying, or they'll lie in bed and want extra tea or coffee brought to them. And they'll want everything brought immediately.

It's difficult for the nurses. On the other hand the conditions and facilities are good. They've always got clean sheets they can put on the beds, and things like that, which is a great help. I don't know what it's like in the rest of the private sector.

But the vast majority of patients, here or anywhere, are basically sensible and grateful. You've got to understand – and it's not just in nursing – that when you first meet a person, nine times out of ten the front they present isn't really them at all. They're either very nervous, which is quite usual here, or they're shy, and they either appear to be grumpy or aggressive, and they're not really like that underneath.

We have the scientific side here, as well as the clinical side, and it's the first time I've worked very closely with medical scientists. They've got a very different attitude. Sometimes I feel they forget they're dealing with human beings. They see the patient as a condition, or a number, or a value.

Certainly the personalities at the top here are quite flamboyant. There's never a dull moment.

AMBITION REALISED

I hadn't abandoned my hopes for the children's hospice, and after I'd settled in here I went to see my solicitor, and asked him how I could start gathering money for such a venture without having people think I was putting it in my pocket. He happened to be a member of Granta Round Table. I'd heard of Round Table, but didn't quite know who they were or what they did. Anyway, he said 'Let me think about this, because I might mention it at one of our meetings.'

I didn't hear any more for six months or so, and then one day I had a call from the Table's chairman-elect, who said he'd like to take the project on as their fund-raising activity during his year of office. So at last, after all these years, here was someone taking me seriously, who thought the scheme might be viable.

Everything's snowballed from there. Without the Round Table and their expertise I wouldn't have known where to start financially, which was the big problem. We launched the appeal 18 months ago, and we're now a registered charity.

We've bought the old rectory at Milton, which is a large, secluded house with a good piece of land. The Church of England let us have it for appreciably less than the going rate. We've got planning permission for an extension, and if all goes well we'll be able to open, with 8–12 beds, toward the end of 1988.

I've put in my resignation here, and I'll be starting work as matron-elect in a couple of months. Until we open I'll be busy with all kinds of planning and organising, and I'll be travelling around East Anglia, or wherever necessary, trying to help GPs and hospitals and nurses and the general public understand what we're aiming to do.

It's perhaps unfortunate that we've had to call it the Cambridge Children's Hospice, because although the word 'hospice' does mean a refuge – a place of rest and shelter – to the general public it means a place to die. But we wouldn't take anyone needing acute care. We're not trying to poach from Addenbrooke's, or anybody else who looks after children who'd benefit from active treatment.

We want to try and provide a haven and a helping hand for those families who've got sadness, and who try to look after a very handicapped child at home without any respite. If they knew there was somewhere they could bring their child for a few days, or even a few weeks (and it doesn't matter how often), whenever things got too difficult, like other children in the family falling ill, they'd be able to cope for the rest of the time much better.

I'd hope to set up a system so that I or another nurse would go and see and get to know the families concerned in their own homes first, so it would be a family affair, and the hospice would be like a home from home, like going to spend a weekend with grandparents or an aunt.

There's been a tremendous response in the area. The local army unit is going to tarmac the drive and re-roof the old stables so that we can use them. But it's a continual grind – trying to get the money.

Not everyone agrees with children's hospices, particularly on the medical side. I'm not sure why. I think some paediatricians think they may lose some of their patients. That's not the idea. We're trying to help the families. We're not trying to encroach on medical care. I hope the doctors will come to understand that they can refer patients to us so that we can help *them* out, as well as the families.

Staffing might be a bit of a problem, because there's already a great shortage of nurses in this area, but we've already got about 350 people on our Friends of the Hospice list, and quite a few of them are nurses, not nursing at the moment because of family commitments, so I hope we can have quite a few part-timers, coming in on a regular basis. They'll enjoy it, and it will help everyone. There's a huge reservoir of nursing skill in this country which isn't being used because there's no opportunity for part-time work.

I'm well aware that this is only the beginning. It's just lucky that I've been able to find other people who are sympathetic and able to help me. It's a dream that looks like coming true.

That doesn't happen very often, does it?

Chapter 10

VIEW FROM THE TOP

Maureen Lahiff is chief nursing adviser to Bloomsbury Health Authority, which has the largest budget of any district authority in the country, partly because it administers two undergraduate and three postgraduate teaching hospitals, as well as a wide range of other services.

She is a married woman and a mother with a whole string of qualifications after her name, including an MSc, and just prior to taking up her present and quite recent post she'd spent a decade as an academic, teaching higher nursing skills and understandings at a poly and the University of Surrey.

Before seeking refuge in academic groves she'd been, **inter** quite a lot of **alia**, a ward sister and a health visitor, and knows all about the rough end of the job.

She's an intellectual with the common touch who clearly revels in authority. Her comments were regularly punctuated by Lord Hailsham-like chuckles at her own remarks.

I'm the person responsible for advising the authority on any matter relating to nursing. I provide leadership for over 3,000 nurses, and I'm accountable for their practice.

I don't manage them, though. Before the last reorganisation my equivalent *would* have done, but the day-to-day management has now been separated from the job of professional supervision. Divisional nurse managers do the day-to-day administration, and they are responsible to general managers, who are usually non-nurses. This separation of professional and managerial accountability has happened within the past 18 months, and its implications aren't fully apparent yet. I think it's workable. Some of my opposite numbers don't.

As I see it, a chief nursing adviser has an enormous job – certainly in a district like mine, which is fairly complex. The Bloomsbury Health Authority was created in 1982 from elements which were previously the responsibility of other districts, and even other regions, and this was done deliberately, because the comparatively small area involved not only provides a wide range of high-quality services, but also has a big commitment to the education of health-care professionals and to research and innovation.

The idea was to bring these activities together under one authority in order to rationalise some of the resources, and make them more cost-effective, instead of having two hospitals 200 yards apart providing exactly the same services. We also need to keep a proportion of our effort as headroom for research, and so on. That's quite a complex agenda, involving a lot of change, and they decided that they did need a full-time nursing adviser. Quite a lot of people in a similar post to mine have to split their time between the advisory role and various executive duties. I have none of those at all.

I'd say 99.9 per cent of the nurses employed within this authority are considered to be professionally accountable to me, and that goes right across the board – community workers, all the acute staff, the postgraduate staff, and so on.

They set this job up as a three-year short-term contract, but when it was offered to me I talked my way out of that straight-away, so I've nine years to go now until I retire. I'm loving it, because I can, I consider, *influence* things. There's so much change going on. We have a major recruitment and retention crisis to be tackled. We have the opportunity to make fundamental changes in nurse education. If ever there was a right moment for somebody like me to come in, it's now. Whether I succeed in handling these problems is, of course, another matter. I'll be very sad if I don't, but at least I'll have had a go.

Many nurses who've stayed in the NHS, and who've had a big managerial role in the past, are very angry and very depressed at the loss of that executive function, and I sympathise with them. If you've had a big chunk of something, and it's been taken away, you've got to work out how to manage without it. Some of them say 'If you're only an adviser, how do you know that anybody's going to *take* your advice?'

Well, I've had ten years in education, and if you've learnt to survive in *that* world, you take that with you wherever you go. I had to run a big multidisciplinary team, with people from the biological sciences and the behavioural sciences and nursing – we had 'em *all*. They weren't even all in the same department. And I had no executive powers at *all*. I wasn't in a line-management relationship with *any* of those members of staff. So you learn how to do it, don't you. I had ten years of learning how to do that kind of thing.

I know that it's possible to develop a power base through one's own credibility, through understanding politics, through understanding an organisation, identifying who your cronies are and who your pals are, who's going to support you, who to feed the material to, all that kind of thing. I say, in effect, to my boss 'I know I'm an adviser, and you don't have to take my advice, but I hope that the way I present it will make you realise you'd be pretty silly if you didn't.' If he decides not to take it, that's OK. He's got the responsibility. He's got the executive role. I don't lose any face over that. I *would* lose face if I hadn't made my case. I'm not going to go and sulk, or anything like that. But it's *lovely* when you're proved right.

The very first thing I disagreed with on the board here was the accommodation business. The DHSS had said 'Sell all your property.' I came in halfway through the affair, and one of the first papers that came to the board in my time was all about how we were going to get rid of a whole lot more property, including nurses' homes.

I was absolutely amazed. I said 'You know we've got a recruitment problem and a retention problem. If we can't offer our people more money, at least we should offer them somewhere to live.' They said 'Oh, well. You don't understand. Region tells us we've got to do more than we're doing.' I said 'This is ridiculous', and in the end they said 'This *is* ridiculous. Tell Region to get stuffed.' Or words to that effect. And in the end it wasn't done.

Afterwards the chief manager said 'Well, at least that might teach us to listen to you.' It's not all bad. You can't expect to win everything, but it's not all bad.

THE TROOPS

Recruitment and retention is our biggest problem. I'm guessing, but I'd say that for 15 or 20 years inner-city hospitals – even the teaching hospitals – have depended on agency nurses for keeping their services afloat, and I think this dependency has been hidden.

There are two reasons why people go into agency nursing. One is the freedom. They don't have to commit themselves to an organisation. They get slightly higher money, and they get the freedom. When they've had enough they can say 'I'll take a few nights off' or whatever. Secondly it attracts a mobile workforce – people who like the idea of moving around for a couple of years, and fancy six months in London, and so on. I don't know the figures. I know we spend a lot of money on hiring agency nurses, and I've some idea of the sums involved now, but we do *not* have data going back over the years.

I'd been away from the NHS until I came back last year, and I was amazed at how poor the data are still. I just couldn't believe it. I said 'I want all the information about recruitment, staff turnover, the reason why people leave, how much staff development they've done – a whole range of things.' And they said 'It's not available.' This was probably partly due to the fact that the authority had only recently been formed from bits and pieces of other authorities, but it was also because the information hadn't been collected very well.

So I don't *know* why nurses leave. I have to make guesses, based on my experience.

I believe a lot of people move out of the institutional setting because the organisation – the hospital structure – does *not* allow enough scope for initiative and creativity, for doing things

differently. A lot of nurses blame that on the nature of the NHS.
I don't think that's so. I think it's rooted in the traditional
relationship between doctors and nurses – a relationship that's
perpetuated by both professions. A sizeable proportion of nurses
move out into private health care, or into the community, where
they find a much freer atmosphere.

We've done a follow-up on the careers of graduate nurses.
A high percentage work in the community. It's because they can
use their initiative. They can think. To a large extent they can do
things the way they want to do them without the great weight of
the hospital hierarchy bearing down upon them.

The graduates come in with a proven ability. Many other people
come in with ability, but they don't know how to use it, and tend to
believe that the established structure is the law. The graduates are
an atypical group, and have encountered some difficulty in making
their way, because they question, and they argue, and they assert
themselves, and that doesn't go down too well.

A majority of nurses have not had the education needed to
allow them to appreciate possible improvements to the situation
they find themselves in, but it dawns on them that there are
other ways of behaving, and less onerous and frustrating ways of
making a living, so they get out, instead of staying in and trying
to change the system.

We don't have accurate figures, but we do know that there
are very large numbers of people who've been trained as nurses
who are now out there doing all sorts of other things. I mean,
the number of times you can hear people saying 'Oh, I used to
be a nurse', 'I'm an ex-nurse.' You never talk about ex-doctors,
even if they're doing something which has nothing to do with
medicine. But if a nurse goes into journalism, say, she immediately
becomes an 'ex-nurse'.

Nurses are still doing a lot of the support tasks that could
be done by other people. They're still doing a lot of form-filling
and errand-running. They're awfully good at stepping in and
coping with all manner of chores when something in the system
breaks down.

We're about to rationalise the pathology services here, so that
some labs concentrate on some tasks and some on others. One of

the consultants said to me 'You know what will happen. If they don't get the computers up and going, and if they don't get the transport organised, it'll be the nurses running around all over the district with the specimens.' I said 'Over my dead body! If the system doesn't work, you find some other way of doing it. You won't use the nurses.'

But traditionally the nurses are expected to jump in and do everything. That's a waste of precious skills. We already have the idea of people called ward clerks to look after much of the paperwork, and in Oxford they're experimenting with people called 'housekeepers', who fill in the gap between the work done by, say, contract cleaners, and what are properly nursing duties. Nurses shouldn't be spending time counting sheets and pillowslips.

The trouble is that we can't compete with other organisations because of the levels of pay in the NHS. You can't pay a ward clerk more than a staff nurse, for example. We've vacancies for ward clerks here, and we can't fill them.

There's a lot more we could do in terms of technological support. Putting all the appropriate office technology into the wards could help a lot. The things that *can* be done by machines *should* be done by machines, and it's the things machines can't do we should really focus on – the personal contacts, the emotional support, the psychosocial things. Those will never be handled by machines – I hope. That's got to be people.

I want to see a major change, so that nursing is no longer a task-centred service, with the juniors getting all the easiest and dirtiest jobs, and the third years getting the dressings and the drugs. I want a patient allocation system, where a nurse, together with any junior assistant, takes over the nursing responsibility for a particular group of patients, and having made the nursing assessment, and having planned the pattern of care, that sticks, barring emergencies, and isn't altered, willy-nilly, by any other nurse who comes in on a different shift.

It's very much like the medical model of working. A doctor wouldn't dream of giving everybody identical treatment. You listen, you take a history, you make an assessment, and *then* you decide what to do. You provide a *decision*-based service, rather than just undertaking a series of tasks.

But as I'm often saying to people, any fool can make a decision. What we want is *quality* decisions. So we're talking about somebody who is knowledgeable, as well as being good at decision-making, and also good at the skills of being a nurse.

We're increasingly recognising that patients aren't just objects that you do things *to*. A large part of the management of health and illness is helping people understand how they can help themselves. Nurses are better placed than doctors when it comes to that.

Doctors and nurses have different but equally important roles.

I'm looking at what nursing's going to be like in ten years time, and I say to the doctors 'Well, chaps, they're either going to be equal partners with you, or we're going to have to manage without 'em.' It will be as simple as that. I really believe that. Either we'll be accepted as equal partners, and we'll get the training needed to fit us for that role, or the doctors will be looking for some other sorts of helpers.

PROJECT 2000

We were training vast numbers of nurses, but the figure's been falling over the past six to eight years as part of a deliberate policy. We started *trying* to do some manpower planning, and asking ourselves how many registered nurses we were actually going to need, instead of just bringing in student nurses in the numbers required to staff the wards. So there's been a gradual shift away from basing the service on student labour, and if Project 2000 is implemented that will come to fruition, and students *won't* be the workforce.

The suggestion is that entry requirements should be widened, not lowered, and there *is* a difference. We've had this very rigid requirement of five O levels, *or* passing a very questionable standardised one-off test developed by the English National Board. So the pressure on UKCC, quite rightly in my view, is for the gateway to be broadened, particularly for more mature people. I've been running a degree course, and I wouldn't dream of applying such a rigid rule. For adults you've got to have as many variations in requirements as there are *people*. What you're saying is 'You prove to me why you should be able to come in and do this course. What have you got to offer?'

I had an enrolled nurse ring me up to ask if she could join my course, but she didn't know if she qualified. I said 'What *are* your qualifications?' She said 'I've got a degree', and I said 'Well, how come you've got a degree, and you're an enrolled nurse?' She said 'Well, I went in as an enrolled nurse, because I didn't have the O levels, and after I'd been practising for a while somebody was a bit rude to me, and said I couldn't do whatever it was because I hadn't got any O levels, and I thought "Stuff that!" and went and got them. And I got a bit carried away, and did some As, and then I got carried away further and did a degree.'

We've got to be *much* more flexible. I subscribe to the American system where, in the better places, you can come in as what we'd call an auxiliary, and you can get right through to the top, and a PhD, or anything else you like to mention. You *ought* to be able to do that if you're willing to apply yourself, and you *have* got the ability. It shouldn't be the structure that stops you. We're a long way from that.

I've some reservations about doing away with the second-level nurse. I think having two levels is feasible in practice if you use your head and think it out properly, and then use your managerial clout and *manage* it properly. We haven't done either of those things. We didn't think it through properly, and we certainly haven't managed it properly, and as a result we've ended up with a whole set of problems, and because we can't deal with them we want to sweep the whole thing away.

I must be in a minority of one, but having looked at the manpower implications of Project 2000 I can see a very good argument for retaining a second level, but having much more flexible routes through from second- to first-level status.

I'm an adult educationalist, and I believe – I've so much hard evidence to *prove* – that a bad performance at school doesn't tell you anything about a person's ability for life. That just tells you about their ability as a teenager. Well, a lot of us were very distracted as teenagers. Life was full of other things.

HOW TO TRAIN A NURSE

I don't think there's one ideal course of training, but I do believe, most firmly, that our training should be like other kinds of further education, based in the college or polytechnic or university. Students *shouldn't* be providing the services.

For me a really good course provides a very adequate educational foundation combined with a wide range of practical experience – not in-depth experience, but just putting toes in lots of water across a breadth of institutional settings.

The health needs of our society and the costs of institutional health care tell us that we've really got to be prepared to work both within the institution and outside it. We've got to get rid of those very rigid divisions, which can mean that people have no idea what goes on outside the building – so that they *do* know how people live, so that they appreciate the environmental factors contributing to ill health. Much more care and treatment could be undertaken outside hospital. We haven't moved into day-care surgery to any great extent, or five-day wards, with patients going home for the weekend. We could do a lot more of that kind of thing. And we need to consider the extent to which patients are kept in hospital for investigation. I can remember being admitted to St Mary's for investigation, and I was there for a week before anything happened at *all*. Well, it still cost them all that money to keep me there.

I think the private sector's teaching us quite a lot, because they *have* to keep things cost effective. So there's an increasing recognition of the need to coordinate tests, so that you bring people in for a day and go through a whole range of procedures, and perhaps don't admit them at all. I think there's a lot of mileage in that. I was absolutely delighted to learn that somebody had done a study showing that some consultants will do things quite differently in the private sector and the NHS. I've believed that for years, but, of course, if you go and put it to them, they'll deny it.

So, yes, much more could be done in the community, and the Project 2000 proposals include giving students a much better grounding in a whole range of factors which are relevant to health and illness in society.

We've recently started a system of having some of our clinical nurse specialists working in the community as well as inside the hospitals. Diabetes nurse specialists, for example, will help patients at home to understand and manage their disease, and will provide specialist support for other community health workers, and will also, hopefully, undertake research. We've been able to show that their work is highly cost effective. There's been a significant reduction in the incidence of diabetic coma, and of other complications, and of re-admissions to hospital.

In the past the traditional attitude adopted by both doctors and nurses was 'Well, you've got a hiatus hernia, and you'll just have to learn to live with it. Go off and do it. Dismissed!' Now we understand that as health professionals we actually have a responsibility to share some of our knowledge about *how* to live with it. A whole range of conditions can be made far less disabling, and be far better controlled, if the patient is told how to cope by somebody with the necessary knowledge. It doesn't have to be a doctor. Doctors are expensive and have other things to do. Nurses have a large role here. That's why they need to be trained in psychosocial skills, and to be taught how to communicate.

The present training of both doctors and nurses has this huge concentration on hospital-based practice, whereas the majority of doctors and large numbers of nurses end up working in the community, and it would be sensible if their basic training took cognizance of that fact. The present system not only gives the training an inappropriate focus, but also makes community work seem like a second-class happening.

I'd have a college of health sciences, and have everybody there – the medics, the nurses, the physios, the whole caboodle. We all need an element of physics. We all need an element of psychology. We all need an element of understanding social policy and organisational structure – a whole range of things. It would do us a lot of good to work together. We're light years away from that.

I don't know how you'd decide what route to follow after the basic training. I guess the choice would depend on rewards and status.

It's not only that, though. There's a key difference between medicine and nursing. Medicine is much more a quick homing in on a specific problem, giving an opinion, and going away again. Nursing is not about a series of diseases: it's about the problems of daily life.

A doctor doesn't say 'OK, you've got your leg in plaster. How are you going to keep yourself clean?' But for a nurse that *is* the key problem. It's that teasing out of what nurses always do and nobody else ever does.

One of the reasons why nursing is beginning to flourish in its own right is because there's been a whole neglected knowledge base which doctors haven't had time to address. Doctors haven't *done* massive research into pressure areas, or nutrition. Doctors are only just discovering nutrition. The big advances in nursing research have been in areas like fluid balance and incontinence and pressure areas, and a whole range of issues which are very important to the welfare of patients but which doctors have left on one side because they've been too busy with other things.

If you've had an anaesthetic and are unconscious, it's the nurse who'll be concerned about whether you can breathe, whether your airway's being maintained, or whether you're being damaged in any way when you're out of the theatre and the anaesthetist isn't there. Having someone come and wash you every day is rather different from having a doctor come and look at you very briefly, and go away again, however intimate that look might be.

The medical relationship is a more distant relationship. Nursing has the potential for being a more intimate relationship. There's a very real therapeutic angle to nursing.

MEN VERSUS WOMEN

The women's movement is pretty central to the problem. The traditional medical/nursing relationship has been one of male dominance and female subservience.

One of the reasons for women not coming back into nursing after having a family is that they're *not* prepared to be treated as schoolgirls. We really have to allow women to undertake the responsibility of care without being subservient. Otherwise there'll be less and less school-leavers willing to enter the profession.

I'd certainly call myself a feminist, but not of the extreme kind. I think women *have* been put upon in the past, and I believe the traditional imbalance has got to be redressed. But I like to talk not so much about women's liberation as people's liberation, and if we can get the balance right I would see that as an advantage, not just for women but for society.

Because, just as *women* have been forced into a stereotype, so have *men*, and I don't think that's healthy for anybody. Doctors have been forced into a stereotype of superiority, and for many people that's very hard to live up to, and is quite unreal, and does a lot of damage to private lives.

And I'm afraid all the evidence is that men in nursing subscribe to the traditional attitudes, and quickly get themselves into managerial positions where they're asserting and controlling and so on. That doesn't actually help our cause. I think, in any case, that we won't *get* a lot more men in nursing unless the money gets a great deal better, and if that happened a lot of other things would follow.

I don't regard nursing as a peculiarly feminine profession, but the way it's structured *is* peculiarly feminine. It's structured as a low-paid, anybody-can-do-it, you-don't-really-need-to-be-educated kind of career. It fits all the conventional perceptions of 'women's work' – 'You don't really need to be educated to be a nurse', 'You don't really need to be educated to be a secretary', 'You don't really need to be educated to be a home economist', 'These are all things *any* of us can do.' There's this constant perception of nursing as a very simple job that anybody can do. Well, if that's *really* all it is, don't let's *have* an education. Don't let's *have* a career structure. Just go and haul people in off the streets every time you want them.

Everywhere you go you hear people say of Project 2000 'Oh, we're going to make the nurses too academic.' Well, what does *that* mean? You don't hear it said about men. Is an engineer not an engineer because he started in a university? I always like to cite the example of a really good surgeon, who has to be both a thinker and a doer. He has a fantastic knowledge base, and he can use it on the hoof, because as well as having excellent manipulative skills you need to make good, informed decisions fast when you're actually in among someone's guts. So he has to be a thoroughly practical chap. But does anybody ever say 'Surgeons are being made too academic'?

So why this fear of making nurses 'too academic'? It's all rooted in the gender thing. 'Women can't think', 'You don't need to be able to think to care.' Maybe not, but oh my goodness, the difference it makes if you do.

The majority of patients in hospital today are much older and much sicker than the people who filled the wards when I trained, and it's quite, quite wrong to have *anybody* untrained looking after them. I watched a television programme picturing life in a hospital in Leeds, and we saw these student nurses doing their first day on the wards. They'd just finished their introductory course, and we saw one of them giving an intramuscular injection to a patient – a real live injection to a real live patient – and she made a total pig's ear of it. Then we saw another poor girl, who'd never washed anybody in her life except herself, blanket-bathing a terminally ill man with matchstick limbs. She had *no* idea. I felt ashamed to be a nurse. I really did. That we can actually *let* that kind of thing happen. That is appalling. *I* don't want to be learnt on. Do *you*? I don't say it never happened in my day, but there were a lot more people in bed who were fairly robust. Perhaps we could learn our skills on them without causing too much grief.

If Project 2000 goes through, nurses will be more competent and more mature by the time they have responsibility for patient care. The pessimists say 'Oh, we can't possibly do it, because it will cost too much.' We're just doing the costings now, and I'm praying it won't turn out to be as expensive as the pessimists predict. It *could* be cost effective. If we educate nurses properly, and select them more carefully, and if we give them a really good career structure in clinical practice – if we do all these things it could be *much* more cost effective.

At the moment we have large numbers of nurses leaving the profession either during training or within a very few years afterwards. We should really be saying that people coming into nursing have a 30–40–year career ahead of them. Even allowing for quite a high percentage taking career breaks to start a family, we could still get a much better return than we do at present from the investment we put into training. Given the right back-up from auxiliary staff, we could probably manage with significantly fewer nurses if those we do have are fully competent. Implementing Project 2000 could be cost effective.

We can only guess at what will happen if we don't.

I'm very proud to be a nurse.

And I don't pour out the coffee at board meetings.

Chapter 11

RECOLLECTIONS AND REFLECTIONS

Margaret Starkie, registered nurse and midwife, specialist in cancer care, and sometime sister-tutor.

When I trained we regarded doctors as God, which was strange, because we regarded medical students as complete morons. And how the transition occurred, none of us knew, but it was sudden omnipotence overnight.

Everything stopped on the ward when the consultants did their rounds. We were shown training films. One scene pictured the ward sister and a student nurse standing to attention while the consultant bent over the patient, and showed how you should spread your weight on your feet, even while standing at attention, so that you didn't get backache, and didn't get blood pooling in your legs. I found this incredible.

Later on, when I was a sister at the Middlesex, the chief cardiologist, who was extremely well-known, actually had the porters go out and stop the traffic in Berners Street while he did his ward rounds so that he could listen to people's hearts. I always felt that if he needed to do that either his hearing wasn't very good or his stethoscope wasn't too marvellous. But I'm sure it was just an affectation, to add to his majesty.

I have strong memories of being told by sisters to straighten the counterpanes because the consultant was about to do a round, when what we should have been doing was making the patient more comfortable.

I felt a tremendous rebellion against that kind of thing, because it could be in nobody's interest to have the doctor so set above everyone else. There could be no discussion. Things began to get much softer soon afterwards. They were tending to appoint younger consultants.

I went to the Royal Marsden for their cancer nursing course, as it was then called. That was extremely interesting because they were at the forefront of many developments which were new at the time.

They were just beginning to use methotrexate for the treatment of chorionepitheliomas, and it was a great joy to see these girls, many of whom were very young indeed, being cured of a cancer which a few years before would have killed. We were also using chemotherapy for leukaemia, which was changing the course of the disease.

I enjoyed the technical side of it – the use of ionising radiation and the methods of diagnosis. I did a lot of extra work and learning on the use of isotopes.

One of the nice things about oncology nursing was that the patients stayed in a reasonable length of time. In general surgery the average stay is about eight days, but my patients would come in for a six-weeks' course of treatment, and so we got to know them very well.

We obviously had a lot who died. Many came in for a course of treatment and then went home, and then they'd come back, not quite so well, for another course, and go home again, and then come back and die. That was just one of the things you had to accept about that sort of work.

Later I had a cancer ward of my own at the Middlesex. We had a lovely woman with carcinoma of the tongue. She was a long-term Soho prostitute. She had dyed red hair and was an absolutely fantastic character. I'd say she was probably a psychopath. She was a pathological liar, I know that. She'd been brought in from Holloway Prison where she was serving a sentence for shoplifting, and she had a warder to sit with her all the time. What they thought she was ever going to get up to, I can't *imagine*. Anyway, she had 15 radium needles put in her tongue. I remember the number, because we had to count them every day. The needles had to stay in for six days, which was a terribly uncomfortable business, and she had to have all her feeds through a straw.

On the third day I rang up the governor of Holloway and said 'Look. You can't leave this prison officer sitting here all day long because she'll get too high a dose of radiation, and this poor patient's not going to be able to *go* anywhere while she's got the needles in.' So the warder went away and left us with this prisoner, and we rather forgot she *was* a prisoner, and forgot to tell Holloway that she'd had her needles out and was going for convalescence at our recovery unit near Kenwood up on Hampstead Heath.

She immediately absconded and went back to her old tricks, but found that prostitution and a sloughing carcinoma of the tongue didn't go well together, and she appeared on my ward a few days later and said 'Please will you help me?' So we took her in and told Holloway, and they decided that if she could be a good girl she could go back to convalescence, and they'd send a warder out there. I'm sure the prison officer enjoyed it, because it was a lovely place.

We had a woman with polycythaemia vera, when the bone marrow produces too many red cells, and the treatment involved injecting radioactive phosphorus directly into a vein, which damps down the cell production. So then, of course, *she* became radioactive. Unfortunately she had a massive blood clot in her brain, and died, and there we were with a radioactive body. The mortuary staff wouldn't take it. She sat there in my side-ward for three nights. We weren't allowed to do last offices, and the relatives weren't allowed to see her, or anything. She just had to sit there while the radioactivity decayed. It was awful. It was bizarre. And then they brought up a lead-lined coffin, and put her in that, and she was taken away.

It was an interesting time.

You got used to death. You do get hardened. We once had three deaths on Christmas Day, and I sat in the office and smoked cigarettes and drank half a bottle of gin. It didn't exactly do me any good at all.

I *smoked* when I was a ward sister. It's an awful thought, because we had lots of patients with carcinoma of the lungs. But I and another sister who had an equally tough ward often said we'd have become alcoholics if we could have afforded it.

You *do* get used to death. The most difficult things are trying to explain to people why their relatives have died when they weren't there, and trying to keep all the student nurses and domestics happy when you've had a spate of deaths.

I think everybody thinks that death is beautiful, and it's *not*.

Doctors don't have the caring role that nurses have. It's a completely different role. And although I enjoyed being able to *look* at diagnosis and therapy in a great deal of detail, and read a lot, I wouldn't like to have it imposed upon me. I liked nursing patients.

There's no greater joy than giving somebody a bed bath, and leaving them comfortable and clean and happy. When I was a tutor I thoroughly enjoyed teaching on the ward and doing the physical nursing with a nurse. This I enjoyed more than anything. It's a completely different world.

I don't see any reason why nurses shouldn't be as *well* educated as doctors, and follow as good and as successful a career path, with as good remuneration in the end.

I was furious when those two people came back from that Beirut camp – Dr Cutting and her nursing partner – and they both got honours. But the doctor got an OBE and the nurse an MBE. I thought 'This is like officers and other ranks.' I thought that was appalling. The hierarchical system where doctors are regarded as very much better than nurses really annoys me.

That's one of the reasons why I was quite happy to come out of nursing. It's one of the things we fought against when we were student nurses, and I really think that now, 25 years later, it shouldn't go on.

Margaret Leader is a practice nurse.

Some patients will come in and they really just want to talk to you. All they want is a listening. Some will ring up and say 'I want an appointment with the nurse.' The receptionist will say 'Well, what's it for?' They'll say 'I don't want to say, but the nurse will understand.'

After you've been with a practice for a time you've built up a relationship with the patients, and probably with a whole family, and with the aunts and uncles and cousins. They'll talk to the nurse, and tell you things which they probably wouldn't say to the doctor.

I've had girls who have come in to me who are pregnant, and they daren't tell their mothers, and they certainly daren't go to the doctor. By talking to them you can just edge them round to seeing the doctor, and they'll go in the end.

———————

People today rely far too much on their GPs. They'll come to the doctor for every little scratch on their finger. Sometimes that annoys me. They can't think for themselves. They can't fend for themselves. I sometimes think that if they had to pay a small fee, that would keep a lot of people away.

Alison Baker is a district nurse.

It's nice to be your own boss. I think that's what I disliked in hospital. I disliked the hierarchy. I disliked the constant harrassment, and the changing around. Everybody seems to be getting at you – whether it's the doctors wanting things, or the sister wanting things, or the auxiliaries wanting support, or the porters wanting to know where someone was or someone's notes were, because they had to go down somewhere.

You're your own boss in the community. You can take one patient at a time, and perhaps devote half an hour to that patient, and talk, and listen. And you can see results, whether it's a leg ulcer getting better or a patient getting his independence back, little by little. Setting goals and actually achieving them.

Bridget Keast-Butler trained as a nurse at the Middlesex Hospital and is now married to an NHS consultant.

I was accepted by St Thomas' Hospital and I turned them down. They didn't like me writing on lined paper. At my interview they said 'Why have you written on lined paper?' I said 'It was the only thing I had to hand.' And if my writing hadn't been so neat, and if I hadn't had the father I had, they wouldn't have looked at my application. Because I'd written on lined paper.

———————

Patients don't know that you're only 18, and they unburden their souls to you. They expect you to know all the ins and outs, not only of their medical problems, but also their emotional problems.

You act it out, or tell them you don't know, and will go and find somebody who does know. But I'm sure that nurses get told an awful lot more than some doctors. Simply because you're always there, and when you're doing things like bed-bathing, and talking to them, they tell you things they might be too frightened to tell somebody else.

Sometimes they want it passed on, and sometimes they don't.

———————

One of the problems in the NHS is that nobody's ever made to think what their actions are costing.

A long time ago I let someone have breakfast who should have been starved, because he was having a barium meal. The consultant said 'Why isn't this chappy having his barium meal?' and I said 'I'm afraid I gave him breakfast,' and he said 'They should charge you £140 for that, because he's staying in this ward for an extra day, unnecessarily.' That *stuck*.

But on the whole people aren't told that what may not be a catastrophic error, but just a human error, due to inefficiency, is actually costing somebody, somewhere along the line, a lot of money.

———————

I don't know that I'd want to go back to nursing now, because it's got very fragmented, and the authority's very much divided, and the whole feeling of a small club has gone.

When we trained, the engineers used to mend the nurses' hair dryers. If you had problems there was always somebody around. The porters came when requested, and if the porters weren't there, the nurses did it. And the ward orderlies were under the control of the ward sister, rather than a supervisor. And when they weren't there the nurses cleaned the wards. This may not be the right thing, but it certainly made you part of a small team. Not everybody likes that as a lifestyle, but those who do had a good time.

I've got friends who've gone back to nursing who are not allowed to pick up this or that because if they do the orderlies will go on strike. It's not part of their so-called job.

A lot of goodwill has gone out of the NHS.

A nurse, whatever she feels, is never a boss. She'll never be a boss, because ultimately it's not her who has to take the decisions.

Nursing is very much a service industry, and if you have *too* high qualifications then you're going to want to be the boss. But nursing isn't a boss job. You're always under the authority of the doctor. In the end the doctor's going to do the cutting along the dotted line, and the doctor's going to carry the can if things go wrong.

John Keast-Butler is a consultant ophthalmic surgeon.

One of the best theatre staff nurses we've ever had was an SEN. Absolute perfection.

She gave up eventually. I think she was quite well fulfilled, in that she wasn't desperately ambitious, and wasn't particularly sad that she could never become a theatre sister. But it was frustrating for *us* in that she had more than enough ability to be in a higher post than she was. But she'd no prospects of getting there.

Certainly one wants to encourage people to go into nursing, and terribly high-powered qualifications aren't really necessary. It's the same with medicine. It's terribly difficult to get into medicine, and there's a lot of concern that the four As and a B-type person who's getting in won't necessarily turn out to be a very good doctor.

There *are* some people who are very clever who can also be very human, but a lot of very clever people find it difficult to understand more normal mortals.

A long time ago, when I was a house physician working in a huge hospital with well over 1,000 beds, the person in charge of the men's medical ward was the first male nurse I'd ever worked with. He was the most astonishing person, and it was the most amazingly well-organised ward I've ever worked in.

I think he was ex-forces, and he wasn't like a lot of male nurses. He was definitely *not* homosexual. He was married, and his wife was also a nurse. He was physically a huge chap, and he was a huge character as well. He got tremendous loyalty from the staff. He had an amazing ability to sort patients out.

His office was at one end of the ward, and he always made quite sure that all the really sick patients were put into the bay opposite his office door. He seldom seemed to go out of his office, except to play cards with the patients, but he knew everything that was going on. And he had complete control over the female nurses who worked for him. There were never any arguments.

And he was an extremely intelligent man. He always read the *British Medical Journal* and the *Lancet*. They came to him before they went to the library. So he was able to ask very awkward questions of the medical staff when they did their ward rounds, because, before 11 o'clock, he'd read both journals from cover to cover, and remembered everything.

In a way he was a bit vindictive. If he didn't like a patient, he'd get shunted down to the far end of the ward.

And I was quite amazed, because I'd been brought up in a teaching hospital where all the nurses were female.

He was one of the most impressive ward sisters I've ever encountered.

I was brought up in the days when the operating list went on until the last patient had been operated on. No questions were ever asked about putting patients off until the next day because the list was running late. You just carried on until you'd finished. The medical staff assumed that everybody else would carry on.

There was no fiddling around. The scrubbed nurse wouldn't suddenly change halfway through the operation because it was the end of her shift.

But when I became a consultant, and after I'd been here a week or two, I was hauled over the coals by the out-patient sister. She complained that my clinics were going on too long, and that made the nurses late off duty. So I said 'What am I supposed to do? Short-change the patients, or deal with them properly?' She didn't have too much of an answer to that, but it was obviously very, very unpopular to run over time.

It's now very counter-productive to try and run over time in the operating theatre. It causes terrible ructions with the more senior staff. You're accused of ruining morale, so you tend not to do it.

That's something that *never* used to happen.

I think there are lots of troubles looming. The nurses are leaving in droves. We're understaffed. They *are* underpaid for what they do, and they find it very difficult to work out how they'll *ever* get paid a reasonable wage without striking, which is very much against their tradition, because they *care* about people.

Maggie Lyne is a chief nurse adviser and personnel director with the Ealing Health Authority.

The camaraderie within nursing is second to none. It's quite phenomenal. It's one of the most social worlds around. I think that a nurse's feeling of well-being and worthwhileness on this earth is quite tremendous, even although you feel quite desperate at times because you can't do this, that, and the other thing.

I went through a period of feeling a bit ashamed at not contributing to the wealth of the nation, in the sense of manufacturing, or that kind of thing. That was early on in the Thatcher government. It was the standard thing then. Unless you were producing, you were worthless. And I'm a Conservative, and I believed that. But I thought it through and lost that feeling fairly fast. We're caring for the people who *do* create the wealth. We're helping other people to develop their energies.

I believe in the NHS. There's a lot more we could do if we could get rid of some of the constraints. There are some bloody marvellous people in it. I really do believe in the right to health without payment. It's a basic human right. I was looking at the way things are run in the States a year or so ago, and I couldn't believe it. No cash – no service. No Blue Cross insurance – no service.

———————

Mrs Thatcher made a lot of statements about too much administration and not enough management in the NHS. She was implying that only the wallies of the world go into the NHS. All the junk brains of Britain were in the NHS. So let's screw 'em. Get more management in there. Chuck in a few outsiders. Chuck in the odd brewer. Chuck in the odd ex-colonel, or whatever. Show 'em how it's done. And all the outsiders have left now, practically. There are a few left.

In terms of the management of change it was a stupid thing to do. She should have said 'Where are the stars we've got inside? How can we give those people greater opportunities, and liberate the talent they've got, and get rid of the suffocation the system creates right now?' I don't believe we do have competent management. Our management philosophy should be that our job is to care for people. Patients are people. Staff are people. *Managers* are people. If we don't care for the staff, we're not going to get good patient care.

We're not examining the conditions under which nurses work. We don't look at the kinds of clothes we give them to wear, the times they start and stop work. What's it *like* when they're short-staffed and are landed with even more dependent patients who can't speak English? Who's looking at the number of people who are dying on that ward in the space of a week? All the desperate things that happen, and which have a substantial effect upon morale.

Our ultimate resources are human resources, and yet we're finance-led in everything. We should be *people* managers, maximising the *capacity* of people and unlocking their potential.

We have 4,000 employees here – 4,000 brains, 4,000 families, 4,000 dreams. And yet we call them '4,000 full-time equivalents'. They are 4,000 Marys, Joes, Johns, Lizzies, or whatever, with all their hopes and aspirations. Even simple things like knowing their names are important.

I'm chairing a group for the regional health authority at the moment, seeking opinions right across the board concerning issues which affect their performance at work, and what they'd change if they had the power. What single most important thing would they want shifted? The RHA decided to invest in that, and not before time.

More people leave nursing than any other profession, and we need to know why.

You have some physicians and surgeons in the NHS who have the lousiest manners that you ever came across. They've been to the best public schools and the best universities. They've had the best education money can buy.

They go to Harleystrasse and they are charm itself, as though they were treating the Queen of England. Then they walk into an out-patient department and they scream and they swear and they shout and think of their NHS patients as 'council house tenants'. Their private patients are treated as 'home owners'. Human beings are devalued in the eyes of some professionals because they're being treated in the NHS. I think it's degrading in the extreme.

I do not believe that doctors in the health service – particularly consultants – should have contracts allowing them to do private and public work at the same time. The NHS is being taken for a ride by a lot of them.

At the moment we have huge areas of overlap between the various health professionals. The country cannot afford to have so many different health professionals, and neither can the clients.

If somebody's ill in a family home, who do you have coming through the door? Your GP. Maybe some kind of hospital doctor like a psychiatrist or a geriatrician on a domiciliary visit. A community psychiatric nurse. A health visitor. A district nurse. Uncle Tom Cobbleigh and all. Yet there are common areas which any one of those people could do without anyone else being present. But we have this ultra-specialisation.

We need a corps of specialists who can advise and support other people, but not do their work for them.

I'd like to see all the national bodies that regulate the health professionals getting together and saying 'These are the health needs of the country. How are we going to meet them?' We've got to see that medicine, nursing, and whatever, is geared to primary health care – to community care – instead of concentrating on episodic hospital care, critical though that is.

We're going to need more care than cure in the future. I'd like to see a core health professional, trained in a college where everybody going into health care shares a common foundation course. They shouldn't be attached to a hospital, but they should have access to *all* the services – social services, community care, the voluntary services, hospitals – wherever the work is being done. That way they'd get a feel of what the world is all about. Afterwards they would stream off and specialise in medicine, or nursing, or whatever.

There's never been a greater need than now for health workers to address themselves to the needs of society, rather than to the interests of their own particular branch of the trade. I'm asking for generosity, and even for the death of my own profession, as some people have said to me.

We're light years away from that.

We need to remember that nursing is a service. It's not an end.

Chapter 12

PROBLEMS AND PROSPECTS

Nurses spend a great deal of their time dealing with patients who have been laid low or are dying as a result of smoking, and so, just like doctors, they know very well what addiction to the evil weed can do. Most doctors have kicked the habit. Many nurses haven't — and that includes some of the most senior and sagacious that I came across. Remember the retired sister who said, perhaps only half-jokingly, that she and a colleague would have become alcoholics if only they'd had the money?

One or two of my respondents surprised me by the bitterness with which they spoke concerning the personal failings and inefficiencies of many of their colleagues, and Sue Waite, the hospice matron, gave the impression that one of her most tiresome tasks was striving to keep the peace among her staff.

These are all signs of stress, and the last is particularly interesting, because internecine strife is something that occurs when a group feels oppressed by circumstances beyond its influence and control. The members turn to blaming one another for their discontent.

And yet all the nurses I've chatted up quite obviously love caring for their afflicted fellow creatures, and derive enormous satisfaction from being able to improve their charges' lot, or from simply providing comfort and support when no improvement can be made, and this most nurses have the opportunity of doing every day of their working lives, for that's what nursing's all about.

Many of the world's workers labour purely in order to earn a living, and those of us who actually enjoy the daily round, and marvel at being paid for doing what we want to do, think of ourselves as privileged. A nurse would seem to be a member of this lucky portion of mankind.

In a recent survey conducted among its members by the Royal College of Nursing, just over half of a 1,000-odd quizzed said they were considering abandoning the trade, but of these only 3 per cent said it was because they didn't like nursing. So why are they leaving in droves? Why are so many women, who've devoted so much effort to qualifying themselves for a job they want to do – for a vocation (and nursing *is* a vocation, or it is nothing) – opting out?

As Maureen Lahiff of the Bloomsbury Health Authority pointed out, nobody actually *knows*, because, amazingly, very small effort has been made to find out. (*There's* modern management for you.) So we have to guess, and rely on anecdotal evidence and the results of the very few small surveys that *have* been done.

Well, it looks like stress. But *why* is there stress?

In the first few weeks of 1988 the *British Medical Journal* carried a series of six excellent articles, followed by a leader, all written by Tony Delamothe, the journal's assistant editor, on the theme of nursing grievances. This, of itself, was a remarkable happening, because, up until very recently, doctors and doctors' journals have paid scant regard to nurses, accepting them as a useful and natural part of the medical scene but rarely bothering to pause and consider what kind of creatures they really are.

Tony Delamothe talked to a number of nurses, just as I have done, and his findings and conclusions very much match my own, so much of what follows echoes the content of his admirable report. I have also used some of the facts and figures he collected, and have found it quite impossible to avoid repeating some of his insights and ideas.

Right, then, why *is* there stress?

POOR PAY

Poor pay is the most obvious target for blame, and it may be an important cause of defection, but it may also be that if nurses were suddenly, tomorrow, paid as much as policemen or hospital officers in the prison service, they'd *still* be leaving in droves. I was impressed by the witness of nurses fondly remembering their training two or three decades ago, when they were paid no more than pocket money. *But they were well looked after.*

The assumption in those days was that the majority of nurses were just passing the time until they got married, or that if they weren't going to get married, and stayed in the profession, they were spinsters, without dependents, who didn't *need* much money. There was no need to make nursing a financially-rewarding career. When the young ladies left, to have their bread bought by their husbands, there were always plenty more to take their place.

Times have changed. Nobody goes into nursing to make money, but nurses do need to earn enough money to survive. A recent study has shown that about a third of all nurses have one or more children living at home, that more than half are supporting another adult, and that seven out of ten nurses provide more than 40 per cent of their household's income.

One of the hopefuls I spoke to at the nursing fair said she wanted to go to the States in order to let her children get a decent education, which she didn't believe they had a chance of here — not on her wages. (She didn't reckon much to her local state schools.)

So any idea that nurses only need to be paid enough to let them buy toothpaste and tights is hopelessly old-fashioned. Nurses need a living wage, just like the rest of us. Money does count, even though it may not always be the prime consideration.

TOO MUCH TO DO

In defending her administration's support for the NHS, Mrs Thatcher has constantly quoted figures showing how many more patients are going in and out of hospital each year. There's a great increase in 'productivity'.

Is there?

The nursing administrators I've spoken to say that nobody knows what the figures mean. How many patients are discharged too soon, so that they have to be readmitted? Nobody knows. Nobody has any idea whether the present rapid turnover is, in fact, cost effective.

What nurses *do* know is that this hectic pursuit of 'numbers' is killing them. Tony Delamothe quotes a sister.

'Every day we had too many patients for the empty beds available, so the routine admissions would be sent home — sometimes up to three times. Doctors discharged patients too early in order to get empty beds, but patients would come back again, and have to be readmitted.... Sometimes we would have three patients in one bed within a shift. A miscarriage in the night would go home at 8 am. Then an extra day-case patient would be put into the bed. The waiting-list patient who came to the ward at 10 am would wait until 5 pm. (And if the day-case patient bled, the waiting-list patient went home and came back next morning starved for a major operation.) It was like a factory. The nurses were literally running, at times we used to be so busy.'

Another Thatcher initiative, aimed at increasing 'efficiency' (that is, 'saving money'), was a 1983 directive that health authorities should provide cleaning, catering and laundry services through a system of competitive tendering. A hospital's own existing departments could bid for the jobs, but so could outsiders, and, inevitably, the cheapest bidders have usually won the contracts.

But to cut charges and still make a profit the contractors have reduced the workforce, taken on part-timers, and generally given their employees a poor deal. So in many hospitals essential tasks are being undertaken by overstretched, disgruntled workers with no commitment to the institution or the job. Often standards have fallen to deplorably low levels, with dirt abounding, meals arriving late, and laundry deliveries delayed.

Who carries the can? Why, the nurses, of course. Perhaps trekking to the kitchens to try to rustle up some food, or touring other wards to try to borrow linen or bits of equipment in short supply, or mopping grimy floors.

Here's a wry but typical complaint from Emma Elliott, a fourth-year nurse undergraduate at Leeds Polytechnic.

'There are no teaspoons on the ward. So you give this patient a boiled egg, and there's this great big spoon, and he can't get it *into* the egg. Have you ever seen an NHS boiled egg? It's the smallest you can get hold of.'

Funny? Yes — but harassing as well.

Because of the pressures, more nurses go sick and more leave, which makes things worse for those who are left. They have to do overtime, and they have to work with agency nurses, who may be excellent creatures, but who may have to be shepherded around.

Officially overtime is paid at time-and-a-half during the week and double-time on Sundays, or time off is given in lieu of cash. But the authorities have found cunning ways of avoiding this extra expense. Many hospitals insist that permission for using nurses on overtime must be sought in advance, and if, as commonly occurs, the sister asks a girl to stay without prior notice, because of a sudden rush of work or because somebody hasn't turned up, she can only be offered time off in compensation, and no extra money. But if she takes that extra time off she knows it means more work for her already-overstretched colleagues, so she doesn't insist on her 'rights'.

Most nurses do a couple of hours or more of *unpaid* overtime each week. One slightly bloody-minded SEN I interviewed said she always refused unless the sister was the kind who rolls up her sleeves and mucks in with the workers when the going gets tough.

The most absurd and cynical cash-saving exercise involves the use of agency nurses. I have said that these 'temps' may need to be shepherded around, but some don't because they are actually sent by the agency to work in their own hospital or even their own ward. Agencies are only allowed to pay their girls the standard rate for the job. It is therefore cheaper for hospitals to hire their own staff for additional hours of duty through an agency – the agency's commission of 10–12 per cent adds less to the bill than the cost of employing that same girl at overtime rates.

In one survey nurses put poor staffing levels above poor pay in their list of the causes of discontent. They may be poverty-stricken, but are more worried by the fact that they can't do a proper job of work.

DEATH

We have already referred to the Bedford study which suggested that coping with death may be the most important single cause of stress among hospital staff.

Margaret Starkie said 'You get used to death.' She clearly wasn't 'used to death' on that Christmas Day when she sat in her office smoking and getting through half-a-bottle of gin. And Margaret Leader, the practice nurse, told me she thought that having to cope with the dying and their relatives would be the main thing that would deter her from going back to hospital work.

Perhaps nurse managers and doctors and administrators should pay far more attention to providing support and counselling for the young girls who are too often thrown in at the deep end and left to deal with harrowing scenes and unfamiliar grief.

Several of my respondents remarked on the fact that doctors seem particularly shy of death, seeing it as a defeat in their crusade against the grim reaper and his wily ways. They walk past the beds of the dying. They stop talking to them. That doesn't help the nurses much.

No – I don't believe anybody ever genuinely 'gets used to death'.

ACCOMMODATION

Maureen Lahiff managed to stop her authority selling off nurses' homes in Bloomsbury, but elsewhere a great deal of subsidised accommodation has disappeared. Marie-Louise Curtin, the graduate sister at Atkinson Morley's, is lucky to share a pleasant flat in the hospital grounds, for which she has to pay a 'realistic' rent. Marian Sharpe, the SEN, can only share a private flat in Putney because her parents helped her finance the deal, and she has to do quite a lot of moonlighting to meet her costs.

Most nurses have to find their own accommodation. If they want to live near the job in an inner city they can probably only afford a pretty humble home. The alternative is to move further away and face expensive journeys at difficult times of the day and night using increasingly inadequate, and, indeed, increasingly dangerous and unpleasant, forms of public transport. Few can afford a car. Many look for work near a place where they *can* find somewhere to live, so that the task of staffing inner-city hospitals becomes even more difficult.

Selling off nurses' homes and houses has been one of the sillier 'economies' dreamed up by our present governors.

Policemen are provided with rent-free accommodation, or else receive a substantial annual rent allowance. Why can't nurses have the same?

MANAGEMENT

For over 20 years, successive governments have tinkered with the organisation of the NHS, with no very obvious benefits to the customer, but with a marked and entirely unhappy effect upon the morale of the labourers in the medical vineyard who are often unsure of their place in the scheme of things and uncertain of their future.

The nurses who can remember them regret the passing of the old days when matron was queen, with sole authority over her domain. You knew where you were and who to go to in time of trouble. That happy state of affairs was far too simple for the bureaucrats and planners, who 'improved' it out of existence long ago.

In the last reorganisation but one, which happened in 1974, so-called consensus management was born, with an administrator, a treasurer, a medical officer and a nursing officer sitting together and striving to agree on how things should be done within their health district. A thumbs-down response from any one of the four could block the contrivings of the rest. The matron, with her Florence-Nightingale-type autonomy, had disappeared, but at least a nurse retained a powerful presence in the management team.

Then, in 1983, another stir-up took place, with the creation of general managers who were given the responsibility for taking decisions at regional, district and unit level. Some doctors, treasurers, and even a few nurses, have been appointed to these posts, but the majority are occupied by former administrators, and quite a few incumbents were imported from outside the NHS (the 'odd brewers and ex-colonels' dismissed by Maggie Lyne of Ealing with such scorn).

As a result of this change in the hierarchy, many nurses now feel that their interests are not adequately represented and their problems not properly comprehended along the corridors of power. Every district general manager does have a nursing adviser, like Maureen Lahiff and Maggie Lyne, attached to his HQ staff, and Mrs Lahiff eloquently described her technique for making her presence felt and her views stick. That's all very well, but they *are* only advisers, and whether they are effective in championing their nurses' cause will depend entirely upon the skill with which they can manipulate the thinking of their boss, and on how far the boss is willing to be manipulated. A lot of nurses don't believe this is good enough. The nursing adviser no longer has an automatic right to a place in the management team. The Royal College of Nursing estimates that about one-third of districts lack an effective nursing voice.

One particularly unfortunate arrangement (and one which clearly underlines the government's primary aim) is that general managers can earn an annual bonus, the size of which depends upon their 'performance'. What this really means is that the more money they can save, the better off they are themselves. And, since nurses' salaries constitute the largest single item on their list of recurring costs, they are tempted to cut staffing levels, and have often done so to the extent that services break down. It would be quite unjust (wouldn't it) to put this down to personal greed. Let's say it happens because the new-style managers often haven't much of a clue about what goes on in the wards, and that if they'd had a nurse at their side possessed of adequate clout they'd never have got away with it.

Martin Latham, a nurse undergraduate at Leeds Polytechnic, cites less disastrous but none the less disturbing examples of harm arising from this cutting-the-cost-must-be-our-main-aim philosophy.

'There are two types of sets for giving intravenous fluids. One is 10 pence cheaper than the other. But the cheaper variety is quite dodgy, because you can't alter the rate of the drip very easily, and they have a habit of going off on you. You have to keep a constant eye on them, otherwise an extra litre of fluid can be going in without you noticing. Yet the management will buy the cheaper kind. It's cheaper, so that *must* be a better deal. They don't understand the knock-on effect.

It's the same with catheters. They buy the cheaper versions, and don't understand that these are more liable to cause a bladder infection, which is going to cost £80 a day to treat.'

A major complaint against the elaborate management hierarchy devised by businessmen and civil servants, and apparently loved by politicians, is that in order to gain promotion and earn a good salary not *too* far below that of a fairly junior policeman, a nurse has to stop nursing. She has to become a desk person. This leads to a wicked waste of expensively-trained talent, and deprives active nurses of the experienced leadership, and patients of the experienced care they need.

It has now been decided that nurses with special clinical skills and post-registration certificates shall indeed receive a little extra cash, but that's still a long way from according the skilled practical nurse the same recognition as that given to skilled practical doctors.

Nurses go into nursing because they want to nurse.

Young Martin Latham said 'The day they offer me a manager's job I shall retire.'

STATUS

Nurses feel undervalued. As Maureen Lahiff put the matter, nursing is perceived as 'women's work' and it's widely believed that 'You don't really need to be educated to be a nurse.' That this perception of nurses is shared by many doctors (who should know better) is confirmed by the conversations I've had with graduate and undergraduate nurses, who've found that their relationships with doctors become much easier once their academic status is made known. The doctors suddenly start talking to them as though they were intelligent fellow professionals. The fact that they hadn't been doing so before is a pretty good indication of their opinion of the intellectual capacity and position in the scheme of things of the 'ordinary' member of the tribe.

This stereotype image of the nurse as a subservient female, obediently filling the natural role of her sex as universal mother and caterer to the needs and comforts of the dominant male, is widely perceived. Even the far from subservient Maggie Lyne, when asked what she thought of male nurses, replied 'This is a kind of childish notion I have, but in the main I feel that nurses should be women and that doctors should be men. I mean, it's not a *manly* profession, is it?' However, having let that instinctive prejudice reveal itself, she immediately added 'Why do I make that daft statement, when it was monks who started nursing off all those years ago?'

'Why do I make that daft statement, when it was monks who started nursing off all those years ago?'

A subtle indicator of the prevalence within the profession itself of a gut feeling that nursing is essentially 'women's work' is the frequency with which I was told that 'male nurses tend to be gay' – the assumption that to be attracted to the career a man must, surely, be a bit of a woman. I suspect this to be a total myth. No doubt there *are* some homosexual male nurses, just as there must be quite a few lesbian lady nurses, but I don't suppose the proportion of gays to be found in nursing uniform (or, more likely, sitting behind a desk) is greater than that within the population as a whole. Certainly none of the male nurses I met were in the least bit effeminate, and the people who spoke to me about male nurses they'd come across never remembered these actual acquaintances as 'queer'. It's the others 'out there' they hadn't met who were credited with this propensity.

An almost universal response to questions about the lowly status accorded to nurses within the medical hierarchy was the opinion that they largely had only themselves to blame. They haven't asserted themselves. They haven't answered back. They have meekly accepted the position assigned to them by God, society and the doctors.

It is, however, abundantly clear that the worm is on the turn. Nurses are no longer prepared to behave like good Victorian children, being seen but not heard.

STRIKES AND DEMONSTRATIONS

The first-ever nurses' strike was staged for just one night in January 1988, when 37 members of staff at North Manchester General Hospital refused to report for work. The event gave dramatic proof of the fact that some nurses are now ready for open revolt. Those involved were protesting against a government proposal to replace special payments for night, Sunday and bank holiday work by a lower flat-rate supplement for all duties involving unsocial hours. The 'savings' were to be applied to increasing the pay of nurses with special skills. However, a lot of nurses without such skills (and there *are* a lot) would have been a good deal worse off, with a full-time senior night sister losing nearly £40 a week.

To attempt to introduce such a scheme when discontent within the profession, for all sorts of reasons, is so widespread and so well recognised argues an alarming lack of sensitivity and imagination and even common sense on the part of the people responsible for keeping the NHS afloat.

Within 24 hours Mr Tony Newton, the Health Minister, claimed that the strikers had been 'misled' by their union, and gave a pledge that there would be no reduction in pay for existing staff whose working arrangements remained unchanged. In other words the strike, which earned immense publicity, was an instant and complete success. However, a nursing auxiliary, who was not on strike, but who supported her colleagues on the picket line, said it was 'the saddest night I have ever had in a hospital'.

The strikers were all members of the National Union of Public Employees (NUPE). Nurses belong to one of three unions. The largest is the Royal College of Nursing (RCN), with 265,000 members. Next comes the Confederation of Health Service Employees (COHSE) with about 146,000 nurse members. NUPE claims 80,000. The RCN is much concerned with education and generally promoting the profession's skills and standing, as well as negotiating on its members' behalf, but is becoming increasingly involved in politics. It does not admit auxiliaries. The general secretary is a man.

The RCN's rules forbid strike action, and Mrs Thatcher claims that her government established a nurses' pay review body in 1983 and accepts its recommendations in recognition of this fact, but reserves the right 'to exclude from the scope of the review body recommendations any groups that do resort to industrial action'. In fact in two of the four years 1984–7 the government reneged on its side of the 'bargain' by staging or delaying implementation of the annual award.

A second government manoeuvre has been to fund part of the awards from existing hospital budgets, which has resulted in additional cuts in services, so that nurses are put under extra strain, and are even inhibited from demanding as much as they feel they should have.

At the start of 1988 enough RCN members signed a petition to force the college to sound out opinion within the ranks as to whether the no strike rule should be revoked. The results were announced in March, and an overwhelming majority said 'No'.

COHSE once recruited most of its nurse members from the large psychiatric hospitals. However, these are being closed down, and it is now concentrating on attracting community workers. NUPE appeals to auxiliaries and SENs. Both COHSE and NUPE are pretty militant, and are fond of strikes.

The three unions are not the best of friends. Put bluntly, there's a 'class' difference. A recruiting brochure for QUARN officers includes a separate paragraph saying that RCN sisters are encouraged to continue their membership and college activities 'wherever they are serving', but stays silent on the matter of the other two organisations.

For the moment, therefore, over half of all nurses are debarred from expressing their anger and frustration by going on strike, but if they are tried beyond endurance that (for the government) happy state of affairs could end, either by the RCN changing its rules, which seems unlikely to happen, or by its members defecting in droves to one or other of the rival and less restrained workers' guilds.

There is nothing to stop them marching, and waving placards, and telling the Great British Public just what they think of the way their service is being run, and this they are doing with increasing frequency and vigour. Demonstrations by nurses are not a new phenomenon. A rash occurred in 1982, but whereas then the protests were entirely concerned with pay, today they are just as or even more likely to be about ward closures and other sad circumstances of a kind which prevent the protesters from caring for their patients in the way they would wish, and from finding a proper pride and satisfaction in the job.

We have considered the principal causes of discontent. What's to be done about it all?

PROJECT 2000 AND ALL THAT

America, where graduate nurses are the rule, would willingly recruit as many British registered nurses as she could tempt to her shores. Our training is seen as first-rate and its products are considered excellent. That being so, you might think there wasn't much point in changing things. So why bother with Project 2000?

The broad thrust of the project was outlined in the introduction. The UKCC wants to see the creation of a single-level 'registered practitioner' (the council's own term) replacing the present first- and second-level nurses. The registered practitioner would be qualified to assume personal responsibility for the care of her own clients. Beyond that, further experience and education would produce a 'specialist practitioner' who would be skilled in the management of particular kinds of patients such as diabetics or cancer victims, or who would be expert in health promotion or the care of old people within the community, or some other field of nursing practice. The specialist would advise and support registered practitioners, undertake teaching and perhaps be given some management responsibility, but would maintain direct contact with patients.

There would be a 'helper' grade, put to work after a brief training organised by individual hospitals along guidelines provided by UKCC. In its literature on Project 2000 the council has suggested calling these people 'aides', on the grounds that the label 'is simple', and 'conveys the notion of being a helper and not a practitioner'. Better still (in the council's view) 'There is even a chance that, being short, it may actually pass into everyday use and put an end to the indiscriminate use of the term "nurse".' *That's* a revealing comment.

Registered practitioners will start their training with an 18-month common foundation programme which 'must be embedded in health not in illness', and this will be followed by an 18–month 'branch programme', during which the student will concentrate on the nursing of adults, or of children, or of the mentally ill, or of the mentally handicapped. (Originally the council proposed a fifth branch programme for midwives, but, because of a rough response to this idea from the midwifery lobby, has conceded that the present 18–month course of additional post-registration midwifery training should be retained, and that the establishment of more direct-entry midwifery courses should be encouraged.)

The training would produce a nurse who 'will have had less hospital experience than has the practitioner of today', but who 'will be much more aware of the network of caring and support services in the community and of the range of help which may or should be available. We believe this re-orientation of the registered practitioner is the central requirement in producing nursing and midwifery staff geared to meet the health needs not just of today, but of tomorrow and of the years to come.'

Implementation of the project would put an end to the situation currently existing in most NHS hospitals where 'Considerable amounts of nursing care, in some cases the bulk of the direct nursing care, is delivered by students and by those with only a very brief training.' The new-style student nurses would be regarded as supernumeraries when on the wards, and would spend little time on donkey-work. They would be treated much more like other kinds of students, including having to make do on a student grant. To pay them a salary (as at present) would increase the total extra estimated cost of the scheme by well over 40 per cent.

To meet the staffing requirement of an NHS deprived of most of its student labour *and* of its SENs, the profession would need to attract some 10,000 extra recruits of five-GCSE-C-level-or-better calibre each year. Where are they going to come from? The council's plans do allow for 'widening the entry gate' by various so far rather vaguely-envisaged means, but the nursing moguls are insistent that the standard of achievement required for entry into the new one-level sorority should not be reduced below that now required for RGN training. (Perhaps the use of that term 'sorority' is a little misleading, because one tactic suggested for coping with the threatening shortfall is that of attracting many more men into the trade. At present about one in ten nurses is a man.)

The UKCC published its first Project 2000 report in May 1986, and since then the council has been busily consulting everybody with a possible interest in the scheme, including, of course, the government, and has conducted a vigorous propaganda campaign, aimed at recruiting the support of the profession and doctors and civil servants and politicians and anybody else who might help to persuade an economy-minded (many would say mean-minded) administration that the considerable costs involved would be money well spent.

At present prices full implementation of the plan would instantly add an estimated £40 million to the annual £300 million nurse training bill, and the extra funding required would rise to £100 million within a couple of years. In view of Mrs Thatcher's clear disinclination to lavish money on the NHS, a warm government welcome for such an expensive venture seemed unlikely.

However, in May 1988 John Moore, Secretary of State for Social Services, told the Royal College of Nursing's congress at Brighton that the government had given Project 2000 its blessing, and he received a standing ovation from his delighted audience, which was the first time any government minister had earned such an accolade at the college's annual jamboree.

Mr Moore made it plain that in return for giving nurses in training true student status the profession would have to be generous and flexible in formulating entry requirements, so that a wider range of school leavers and also a greater number of mature students could qualify for admission to the craft, with credit being given for such qualities as experience, and it would also have to be possible for suitable candidates from the new caste of 'aides' or 'nurse-helpers' to earn a place in training schools. The changes could not be undertaken overnight, and the question of how the project would be funded was left conveniently vague.

But why this sudden burst of generosity, following so soon upon the 'lavish' pay awards, and the promise to undertake an extensive regrading exercise which would give many hands-on nurses with special skills and experience extra money?

In the first place, of course, the threat of a disastrous nursing shortage in the '90s is now so apparent that even the bureaucrats and politicians have belatedly found themselves forced to acknowledge the need for vigorous defensive measures. We might be able to survive without the NHS, or even with many fewer doctors, but we'd be in bad trouble without the services of a large enough corps of competent nurses. Project 2000 could help nursing to attract and retain more recruits from the evaporating pool of school leavers.

There is, however, a second and less encouraging likely reason for the government's acquiescence to the nurses' plans. Project 2000 could provide the excuse for trying to manage with significantly fewer expensively trained and reasonably paid 'registered practitioners' in both the hospitals and the community, with many more of the much cheaper 'nurse helpers' carrying out, under supervision, a lot of the duties, such as dressings, bathing, administering drugs, and other intimate caring tasks of a kind at present undertaken by fully qualified staff. Indeed, at a press briefing following Mr Moore's Brighton speech a Department of Health and Social Security spokesman revealed that this is exactly what the government hopes to see happen, particularly in the case of chronic invalids, the handicapped, the elderly, and others whose condition is not liable to sudden change.

This admission, together with the news that similar ideas were contained in a report on the future of community care prepared by Sir Roy Griffiths, the government's health service adviser, greatly angered the RCN delegates at Brighton, who rapidly lost the ebullience generated by Mr Moore's original announcement. They passed a resolution deploring the Griffiths report, and Trevor Clay, the RCN's General Secretary, announced that the college would mightily resist any move to boost the proportion of nurse helpers at the expense of qualified nurses. On the contrary, the college believes that the ranks of the qualified must be swelled by many thousands if the needs of a rapidly enlarging regiment of old people for skilled nursing care are to be properly served.

Whether the nursing Establishment can dissuade this or any future government from both saving money and attempting to ameliorate the effects of a skilled womanpower shortage by making a much greater use of unskilled or semi-skilled labour remains to be seen.

Predictably, NUPE and COHSE officials were scornful of the Moore pronouncement, claiming that the government was aiming to get nursing on the cheap. They might well have been right. But the true cause of their discontent was, of course, the fact that the new arrangements would probably denude them of most of their nursing members. They'd be left to represent the aides.

It seems clear that the government's acceptance of the central theme of Project 2000 was an astute political ploy, costing a bit to start with, but perhaps saving lots of money in the end, and that the RCN delegates who stood and cheered John Moore at that Brighton congress didn't immediately cotton on to the possible implications of their 'triumph'.

The war's not over yet.

I see Project 2000 as an attempt to raise the status of the nurse, making her a recognised 'professional', and a creature who would be on more equal terms with doctors, and a person able to command more pay and more respect, and have a louder voice in the land. I don't think it ever had much to do with any genuine or widespread feeling that the nurses we have right now ill-serve their customers.

Nothing wrong with that. Nurses are entitled to fight their corner, and to strive, by all reasonable means, to generate the honour they deserve. But will the implementation of Project 2000 result in patients getting a better deal, which is, surely, the ultimate test to be applied to any proposal for altering the manner in which we organise and deliver health care?

Would a highly educated nurse necessarily be a better nurse? Emma Elliott, at Leeds Polytechnic, told me a nice tale.

'I'd been talking to this auxiliary. We'd been running about, we were really busy, and we sat down to have a drink, and she said "When do you qualify?" I said "Next June." She said "Oh, you're only just a third year." I said "Well, actually, I'm a fourth year, really." And then we got into this degree business, and she said "Oh, you're a degree nurse. I thought you were a *proper* nurse."'

So what is a 'proper nurse'? A 'proper nurse', it seems to me, is a man or woman who has a rare commitment to care, so strong that half-a-million of such people continue to labour in the NHS despite a miserable cash reward and ever-worsening conditions. Certainly nursing needs a good many Lahiffs and Lynes and Curtins and Lathams within its ranks, but it cannot afford to reject the services of tens of thousands of young men and women who may be less academically inclined, or who simply haven't got round to sharing Longfellow's belief that 'Life is real! Life is earnest!' by the time they're 18.

Several of the admirable and clearly invaluable older nurses I have spoken to, who have a long record of meritorious service to their credit, have remarked that they would never have been accepted for training as an SRN if today's entry requirements had been in force in their young days. The highly intelligent and capable SEN, Marian Sharpe, spent much of her time and energy during her last years at school in voluntary nursing service, so that physics, maths, geography, and the rest rather went by the board. She would certainly not have accepted the option of becoming an 'aide', with little prospect of employing her initiative or using her brain or ever becoming more than a ward skivvy, and there must be many, many more like her.

When it comes to serving the needs of the sick and the distressed a good heart and the possession of common-sense can be just as valuable as a good degree, so if Project 2000 is to be a success instead of a disaster it is indeed essential that it should still be possible for men and women with a wide range of academic abilities and paper qualifications (or with no paper qualifications at all) to achieve full nursing status. An unimaginative implementation of the scheme could increase rather than reduce the nurse shortage.

There's another objection. I was often told that some of the most valuable contacts to be had with patients occur during the performance of personal and intimate services, like bathing and feeding.

If the structure of nursing is altered to the extent that students spend little time serving patients in this way, and then, when qualified, are so busy with the more technical and organisational duties of their post that all the chores have to be left to aides, they will at no stage experience such close encounters. They will become distanced from their customers, and a large part of both the satisfaction and the supportive and therapeutic value of the nursing role will be lost. And whatever the UKCC may say, it will be the aide who the patients relate to and call their 'nurse'.

WHAT NEXT?

This last chapter has dwelt largely on the present discontents, and to that extent is not a fair reflection of the conversations I've enjoyed. The nurses I have met were largely concerned to explain and describe the fascination and satisfaction and sheer fun to be had out of their work. Most of them laughed a lot. They didn't spend our time together just rattling off a long list of complaints. But the causes of complaint are there, and to the extent that many can no longer take the stresses and strains of the nursing life, despite its rich rewards.

The implementation of Project 2000 may improve some of the less happy aspects of the nurses' lot, but many will remain, and if we want to be sure of receiving comfort and support next time we're ill, or when faced with the problems of dealing with a fractious infant born to a family desperately striving to make ends meet, or when we are old and none too able to fend for ourselves, or when we are about to die, then the rest of the deficiencies and preventable causes of stress must be tackled urgently.

First of all nurses should be provided with an environment and an adequacy of resources of a kind which will allow them to exercise their skills and fulfil their sustaining role without having to cut corners, or deny their charges the diligent care and prompt attention they should have, and which will put an end to the need for one pair of hands to be constantly striving to cope with a workload that ought to be shared by two. A nurse should be able to go off duty not exhausted and frustrated, but proud and happy in the knowledge of a job well done. Nurses must not be asked to cope with difficulties arising purely and inevitably from a gross underfunding of the organisation in which they serve.

Secondly nurses should be paid and cared for in material ways just as well as policemen, and prison hospital officers, and even doctors, with an experienced sister ranking equally with, say, a registrar of equal age, and so on up the hierarchy. There should be ample opportunity for those who so wish to earn progressive promotion and salary increments during a working lifetime devoted to hands-on patient care. Doctors wouldn't be very pleased if they had to abandon practical medicine and go and sit in an office in order to earn the pay and status of a consultant or a senior GP.

We should adopt the American approach, and actively encourage, and pay for, every nurse able and willing, from the rank of aide or auxiliary upwards, to undergo whatever further education may be needed to take her to whatever position in the profession she wishes to attain. Another sensible American initiative, which ought to be widely copied here, is the effort made over there to cater for the needs of nurses who, because of family commitments, or for any other reason, are willing and able to work part time, or on chosen shifts, but who cannot adhere to a rigid duty rota imposed by somebody sitting at a desk who neither knows nor considers the effect of awkward hours upon the individuals concerned. And how about a generous provision of crèches? Nurses can no longer be treated as creatures with no right to much of a life beyond the 'job'.

Everything that can be done should be done to relieve the nurses of bookkeeping and housekeeping and similar non-nursing chores.

Doctors should be taught – yes, actually *taught* – in their medical schools that nurses are their professional colleagues, providing a different but no less vital part of patient care, and that they are by no means to be regarded or used as mere handmaidens. To help this along, nursing and medical students could well share certain courses of instruction, such as psychology and the structure of the social services.

Finally nurses need to feel that their managers — the people who control the conditions under which they work — truly understand what the job is all about, and have an intimate knowledge and *experience* of the realities of life for the labourers at the sharp end. So I'd bring back the matrons. It's as simple as that.

All this would cost a lot of money — much more than the sums required for an annual 'inflation-plus-a-bit' pay award and a possibly half-hearted implementation of Project 2000. But neither this or any other government is likely to shell out the necessary funds unless subjected to pretty heavy pressure, and the only people who could apply the level of pressure required are the voters.

Tony Delamothe ended his series of articles in the *British Medical Journal* by saying:

'Unless nursing can attract enough recruits from the shrinking pool of school leavers and keep them in nursing, a major crisis will be on us in the 1990s. That is why the nurses' struggle should be the doctors' struggle, too.'

I'd go further than that. I'd say 'That is why the nurses' struggle should be the public's struggle, too.'